Diagnostic Techniques in Urology

Ben Challacombe • Simon Bott
Editors

Diagnostic Techniques in Urology

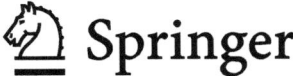 Springer

Editors
Ben Challacombe
Urology
Guy's and St. Thomas' Hospital
London
UK

Simon Bott
Urology
Frimley Park Hospital
Frimley
UK

ISBN 978-1-4471-2765-9   ISBN 978-1-4471-2766-6   (eBook)
DOI 10.1007/978-1-4471-2766-6
Springer London Heidelberg New York Dordrecht

Library of Congress Control Number: 2014957636

Printed on acid-free paper

Springer is part of Springer Science+Business Media (www.springer.com)

*To our patients who provide us with constant
interest and learning*

Introduction and Aims

Diagnosis is not the end, but the beginning of practice. Martin H. Fischer

Clinical diagnosis requires the evaluating doctor to have a clear understanding of both normal anatomy and physiology as well as an understanding of the range of possible pathologies. This allows unambiguous and precise history taking, well directed examination and a clear plan of appropriate investigations to be made.

Urology can be thought of as both a medical and surgical speciality where patients present to a range of different doctors with a wide variety of symptoms. There are a number of nuances to be brought out in a focussed urological history and many important clinical signs to assess. These present the clinician with a significant diagnostic challenge due to the range of possible differential diagnoses and the investigative tests available. Technological advances in recent years have changed the diagnostic algorithms for a number of common conditions.

Within easily digestible chapters, this book aims to succinctly outline the key aspects of the history and examination for each common presenting symptom. It then describes the usual range of investigations and any evolving tests or imaging modalities for each area. It is hoped this book will be useful to both primary care physicians and those working in the emergency department. Medical students and those embarking on a surgical or urological career should also find it of significant benefit.

London, UK   Ben Challacombe
Frimley, UK   Simon R. J. Bott

Contents

Contributors

Nigel Borley, BM, MRCS, MS, FRCS (Urol) Department of Urology, Chelsea and Westminster Hospital, London, UK

Simon R. J. Bott Department of Urology, Frimley Park Hospital NHS Foundation Trust, Frimley, Surrey, UK

Matthew Bultitude, MBBS, MRCS, MSc, FRCS (Urol) Department of Urology, Guy's and St. Thomas NHS Foundation Trust, London, UK

Ben Challacombe, MS, FRCS (Urol) Division of Urology, Guy's and St. Thomas Hospital, Guy's and St. Thomas NHS Foundation Trust, London, UK

Andrew Chetwood, BMedSci (Hons), MBChB (Hons), MRCS Department of Urology, Frimley Park Hospital, Frimley, UK

Prokar Dasgupta, MSc, MD, FRCS (Urol), FEBU Department of Urology, Guy's Hospital Nhs Foundation Trust and King's College London School of Medicine, London, UK

Melissa C. Davies Department of Urology, Salisbury District Hospital, Salisbury, UK

Tamsin Drake, BM, MRCS Department of Urology, Salisbury District Hospital, Salisbury, UK

Nicholas Drinnan Department of Urology, Frimley Park Hospital, Nhs foundation trust, Frimley, UK

James Duthie Division of Cancer Surgery, Peter MacCallum Cancer Centre, University of Melbourne, East Melbourne, VIC, Australia

Ben Eddy, NVQ 1 (Carp), FRCS (Urol) Department of Urology, Kent and Canterbury Hospital, Canterbury, UK

Helen Freeborn Division of Cancer Surgery, Peter MacCallum Cancer Centre, University of Melbourne, East Melbourne, VIC, Australia

Giulio Garaffa, MD, FRCS (Urol) Department of Urology, Urology Centre, Broomfield Hospital, Broomfield, Chelmsford, Essex, UK

St Peter's Andrology, The Institute of Urology, London, UK

Paul K. Hegarty, FRCS (Urol) Department of Urology, Guy's and St. Thomas' NHS Foundation Trust, London, UK

Azhar Khan, MBBS, MRCS Department of Urology, Guy's and St. Thomas' NHS Foundation Trust, London, UK

M. Shamim Khan, MBBS MCPS FRCS (Urol) FEBU Department of Urology, Guy's and St. Thomas' NHS Foundation Trust, London, UK

Clarissa Martyn-Hemphill Department of Urology, Guy's and St. Thomas' NHS Foundation Trust, London, UK

Faith McMeekin, MBBS, BSc, MRCS Department of Urology, Musgrove Park Hospital, Taunton and Somerset NHS Foundation Trust, Taunton, UK

Declan G. Murphy Division of Cancer Surgery,
Peter MacCallum Cancer Centre, University of Melbourne,
East Melbourne, VIC, Australia

Harry Naerger Department of Urology, Frimley Park
Hospital, Nhs foundation trust, Frimley, UK

Ish Naranji Department of Urology, Frimley Park Hospital
NHS Foundation, Frimley, Surrey, UK

Timothy Nedas, MBBS, MSc, FRCS (Urol) Department
of Urology, Guy's and St. Thomas' Hospitals NHS
Foundation Trust, London, UK

Kevin O'Connor Department of Urology,
Royal Melbourne Hospital, Melbourne, VIC, Australia

Anisha Patel, FRCR Department of Radiology,
St George's Hospital, London, UK

Uday Patel Department of Radiology, St George's Hospital
and Medical School, London, UK

Michela Pisani, MD Urology Centre, Broomfield Hospital,
Broomfield, Chelmsford, Essex, UK

Farzana Rahman, FRCR Department of Radiology,
St George's Hospital, London, UK

Nicholas Raison Dept of Urology, Guy's and St. Thomas'
NHS Foundation Trust, London, UK

David J. Ralph, FRCS (Urol) Department of Urology,
St Peter's Andrology, The Institute of Urology, London, UK

Arun Sahai, PhD, FRCS (Urol), BSc (Hons) Department of
Urology, Guy's Hospital Nhs Foundation Trust and King's
College London School of Medicine, London, UK

Jai Seth, BSc, MSc, MRCS Guy's Hospital Nhs Foundation Trust and King's College London School of Medicine, London, UK

Mark J. Speakman, MS, FRCS Department of Urology, Musgrove Park Hospital, Taunton and Somerset NHS Foundation Trust, Taunton, UK

Dan Wood, PhD, FRCS (Urol) Department of Adolescent and Reconstructive Urology, University College London Hospitals, London, UK

Rhana Hassan Zakri, MBBS, MRCS, MSc Department of Urology, Frimley Park Hospital, Frimley, UK

Chapter 1
Prostate Specific Antigen (PSA)

Simon R.J. Bott and Ish Naranji

Prostate Specific Antigen (PSA), also known as kallikrein 3 (KLK3), is a 34kD glycoprotein, encoded by the KLK3 gene on chromosome 19q13. It is a peptidase secreted into the semen by the epithelial cells of the prostate gland. PSA is also secreted in other body fluids including the female ejaculate, where PSA levels are similar to those found in semen; as well as amniotic fluid, breast milk and the secretions from urethral glands. Serum PSA may also be detectable in uterine, breast and lung cancers.

Mechanism of Action

In the prostate, the kallikrein KLK2 inhibits PSA through the action of high concentrations of zinc in an alkaline environment. On ejaculation semen is exposed to the acid environment of the vagina, this reduces zinc inhibition and PSA is activated, the coagulum in semen is liquefied and the spermatozoa is released.

S.R.J. Bott (✉) • I. Naranji
Department of Urology, Frimley Park Hospital NHS Foundation Trust, Portsmouth Road, Frimley, Surrey GU16 7UJ, UK
e-mail: simon.bott@fph-tr.nhs.com

B. Challacombe, S. Bott (eds.), *Diagnostic Techniques in Urology*, DOI 10.1007/978-1-4471-2766-6_1, © Springer-Verlag London 2014

History

PSA was discovered in the 1960–1970s by a number of researchers looking at causes of infertility, for novel methods of birth control and in forensic science for proof of rape in men who may be vasectomized or azoospermic. It was the publication by Tom Stamey, in 1987, of his landmark study looking at PSA in prostate cancer that brought PSA to the attention of the urological community and beyond. Stamey showed that serum PSA increased with prostate tumour volume and stage and was a vast improvement on acid phosphatase. He showed that PSA levels became undetectable following radical prostatectomy and that PSA could be used as a marker for treatment response after surgery and radiotherapy.

Prostate epithelial cells can be stained for PSA using immunohistochemistry. Disruption of the normal epithelium by inflammation causes the PSA to leak into the tissues surrounding the epithelial cells causing a rise in serum PSA. In malignancy individual prostate cancer cells stain less for PSA than individual benign cells, particularly in higher-grade disease. However because cancer contains an increase in the overall number of cells compared with normal prostate the serum PSA level rises.

Diagnosis

Screening

Several large-scale studies have examined the role of PSA to detect prostate cancer in asymptomatic men – population-based screening. The European Randomised Study of Prostate Cancer screening (ERSPC) recruited 182,000 men, aged 55–69, and screened half with PSA every 4 years, the other half acting as a control group [1]. A PSA cut off of ≥3 ng/ml, found in 17 % in the screening arm, prompted a TRUS biopsy. After 11 years' follow-up, men who were screened experienced a 29 % risk reduction in death from prostate cancer, though there was no difference between the groups with respect to all cause mortality. To prevent one death from prostate cancer at 11 years, 1,055 men would need to be screened and 37 prostate cancers detected. Contamination in the ERSPC study was significantly less than a US screening study (PLCO), nevertheless it is estimated that 20 % of those in the control arm had a PSA test per annum.

The Göteborg screening study, which subsequently became incorporated within the ERSPC study, recruited 20,000 men aged 50–64 and screened half with PSA every 2 years [2]. The unscreened subjects were not informed of their participation in a trial and PSA testing was not used routinely so contamination was negligible. After 14 years' follow-up the mortality from prostate cancer in the screened group was half that of the control. Furthermore, half of those who died in the screened group were diagnosed on their first screening visit, many of whom were >60 years. If screening had begun when these men were 50 years, we would expect the mortality rate to fall still further. In this study the number needed to invite for screening was 293 to save one life from prostate cancer, with the number needed to diagnose being 12.

These studies show prostate cancer screening does reduce mortality from prostate cancer, though there is a risk of over diagnosis and over treatment.

In the UK opportunistic screening is recommended, whereby if a man presents with LUTS or requests a PSA test, following appropriate counselling a test should be offered. It is interesting however to note that the PROTEC study has shown that men with a raised PSA and LUTS are less likely to have prostate cancer than those with a raised PSA who do not have LUTS.

PSA As a Predictor of Future Prostate Cancer

Lilja et al. used the stored serum of men enrolled in a cardiac study from the pre PSA era to predict the risk of developing prostate cancer [3]. The serum of men aged 44–50 years was stored. Using the Swedish Cancer Registry 498 men (2.3 % of cohort) were identified who had subsequently been diagnosed with prostate cancer, a median of 18 years after the blood was taken and stored. A single PSA at 44–50 years was shown to significantly predict the clinical diagnosis of prostate cancer and of advanced prostate cancer up to 25 years later [4]. Other studies have used a single PSA taken at age 60 to predict the likelihood of developing prostate cancer metastasis or dying from the disease [5].

PSA range aged 45–50 years	Chance of developing prostate cancer (%)
0.00–0.50	4
0.51–1.00	8
1.01–2.00	20
2.01–3.00	41
>3.0	60

In the future, while more specific markers for prostate cancer are being developed, PSA screening could be refined and tailored to an individual's risk. The Swedish data allow us to predict the development of clinically significant disease, rather than over diagnose insignificant disease as seen in the ERSPC trial for example. Using this Swedish data the following tailored testing could be adopted:

A single PSA check performed at ages 45–50 years can be used to plan the frequency of subsequent PSA testing. A man with a PSA of <1 ng/ml would not need to have another PSA test for 3–5 years and then a third test at 60. If at this point his PSA was still <1 ng/ml (about half of all men) he would need no further tests as his risk of dying of prostate cancer is <1 %. If at 45–50 years his PSA were between 1–2 ng/ml he should have his PSA checked every 2 years during his 50's. If the PSA remains <2 ng/ml at 60 (75 % of all men) he then has a less 5 % chance of dying of the disease and arguably needs no further tests. A PSA >2 ng/ml in the fourth decade should prompt immediate investigation.

This way the majority of men who will not develop prostate cancer only require perhaps 3 PSA tests during their lifetime. Whilst those with greater risk of developing potentially life threatening disease are checked more frequently, reducing the burden of excessive PSA testing and its sequelae as well as cost.

Using a cut-off of 4 ng/mL, PSA has a sensitivity of 67.5–80 % (men who have prostate cancer who have a PSA ≥4 ng/ml), and specificity of 60–70 % (men who do not have prostate cancer who have PSA <4 ng/ml). Put another way, using a cut off of 4 ng/ml will miss 20–30 % of cancers and incorrectly raise the possibility of cancer in 30–40 %. Attempts have therefore been made to try and improve the accuracy of the PSA test including prostate volume based parameters, rate of rise of PSA and the ratio of free to bound PSA in serum.

Volume Based PSA Parameters

Volume based PSA parameters have been evaluated in an attempt to reduce confounding PSA production from benign prostatic hyperplasia (BPH). They include PSA density (PSAD) and PSA transition zone density (PSATZ).

PSA Density (PSAD)

PSAD is serum PSA level per ml of prostatic tissue (PSA divided by prostatic volume). A PSAD of 0.15 ng/ml/ml or greater has been proposed as a trigger for prostate biopsy in men with PSA levels between 4 and 10 ng/ml and a normal DRE, in an attempt to reduce unnecessary biopsies in men with larger prostates. It has also been shown that PSAD is directly associated with prostate cancer aggressiveness. As a result a PSA density of <0.15 ng/ml/ml is the cut-off for suitability for managing patients in part of an active surveillance program according to NICE guidelines (2008).

$$\left(\text{Prostate volume} = \text{Height} \times \text{Width} \times \text{Length} \times \pi / 6 \right)$$

PSA Transition Zone Density (PSATZ)

The transition zone is the major determinant of serum PSA in men without prostate cancer. Djavan et al. found that PSA-TZ was the parameter with the highest overall sensitivity and specificity for prostate cancer detection when PSA was between 4 and 10 ng/ml. A PSATZ cut-off value of 0.35 ng/ml/ml has been traditionally used.

Both PSATZ and PSAD require TRUS volume measurement; this limits their use in routine clinical practice.

PSA Velocity (PSAV)

PSAV is the rate of change of serum PSA. A PSA velocity >0.75 ng/ml per year in at least three PSA tests over a period of at least 18 months may be considered significant. The following formula is used to calculate PSAV

$$PSAV = 0.5 \times PSA2–PSA1/time1 \, in \, years$$
$$+PSA3–PSA2/time2 \, in \, year$$

Vickers et al. showed in a number of studies that PSAV does not predict the outcome of prostate biopsy over PSA alone, nor did it improve the detection of aggressive prostate cancers.

However, the rate of rise of PSA prior to radical prostatectomy does have prognostic value. Men whose PSA rose by ≥2 ng/ml during the year before the diagnosis have a higher risk of death from prostate cancer after surgery than those with a slower rate of PSA rise.

PSA Doubling Time (PSADT)

PSADT is the length of time PSA takes to double in months. At least three PSA results are needed over at least 6 months to determine PSADT.

PSA DT is used in some active surveillance programs and a PSADT of <3 years may prompt radical treatment. PSADT is also used after treatment as a short PSADT (<3 months) predicts metastatic disease, whereas as a PSADT>9–12 months is more indicative of local recurrence.

PSA Free to Total Ratio

The PSA F:T ratio is the percentage of free PSA compared to total PSA in serum. Men with prostate cancer have a lower percentage of total PSA circulating in the free form; hence the ratio is lower in men with prostate cancer than with BPH.

With a normal DRE and a PSA between 4 and 10 ng/ml, the overall risk of prostate cancer is 27 %. This risk rises to 60 % if PSA F:T ratio is <10 % and falls to 10 % if ratio is >25 %. It is important to take in consideration that free PSA is unstable, and therefore serum must be assayed within 3 h or frozen at −20 °C.

Studies investigating variants of PSA in the diagnosis, assessment of cancer aggressiveness and tumour stage are frequently contradictory and seldom outperform PSA alone in well-designed clinical trials.

PSA After Treatment

PSA levels are monitored at regular intervals following treatment. The frequency of monitoring depends on national guidelines and risk group of the patient. The half life of PSA is 2–3 days. After radical prostatectomy PSA becomes undetectable within a few weeks. Follow-up is typically every 3 months for the first year, every 6 months for 3–5 years and annually thereafter. A PSA rise above 0.2 ng/ml during follow-up is generally regarded as evidence of recurrent prostate cancer.

After both external beam radiation therapy and brachytherapy PSA levels are still detectable even after successful treatment. The PSA should fall to a nadir. A PSA rise of 2 ng/ml or greater above the nadir (Phoenix criteria), after either treatment, is considered treatment failure.

References

1. Schröder FH1, Hugosson J, Roobol MJ, Tammela TL, Ciatto S, Nelen V, Kwiatkowski M, Lujan M, Lilja H, Zappa M, Denis LJ, Recker F, Páez A, Määttänen L, Bangma CH, Aus G, Carlsson S, Villers A, Rebillard X, van der Kwast T, Kujala PM, Blijenberg BG, Stenman UH, Huber A, Taari K, Hakama M, Moss SM, de Koning HJ, Auvinen A. ERSPC Investigators Prostate-cancer mortality at 11 years of follow-up. N Engl J Med. 2012;366(11):981–90.
2. Hugosson J1, Carlsson S, Aus G, Bergdahl S, Khatami A, Lodding P, Pihl CG, Stranne J, Holmberg E, Lilja H. Mortality results from the Göteborg randomised population-based prostate-cancer screening trial. Lancet Oncol. 2010;11(8):725–32.
3. Lilja H, Ulmert D, Björk T, Becker C, Serio AM, Nilsson JA, Abrahamsson PA, Vickers AJ, Berglund G. Long-term prediction of prostate cancer up to 25 years before diagnosis of prostate cancer using prostate kallikreins measured at age 44 to 50 years. J Clin Oncol. 2007;25(4):431–6.
4. Ulmert D1, Cronin AM, Björk T, O'Brien MF, Scardino PT, Eastham JA, Becker C, Berglund G, Vickers AJ, Lilja H. Prostate-specific antigen at or before age 50 as a predictor of advanced prostate cancer diagnosed up to 25 years later: a case-control study. BMC Med. 2008;6:6.
5. Vickers AJ, Cronin AM, Björk T, Manjer J, Nilsson PM, Dahlin A, Bjartell A, Scardino PT, Ulmert D, Lilja H. Prostate specific antigen concentration at age 60 and death or metastasis from prostate cancer: case-control study. BMJ. 2010;341.

Chapter 2
Prostate Biopsy and Imaging, and Management of a Rising PSA Post Initial Biopsy

Ben Challacombe

Introduction

Following the discovery of an elevated PSA and evaluation with a digital rectal examination (DRE) a clinical decision needs to be made as to whether further action is required. If there is a suspicion of infective or inflammatory causes for a PSA rise then a further PSA is indicated in 4–6 weeks after appropriate antibiotic treatment. If the DRE is suspicious for malignancy or the PSA seems raised without the presence of infection then further investigations are required. Traditionally this has been in the form of a trans-rectal ultrasound guided (TRUS) biopsy of the prostate. In the last few years further options have emerged with the addition of trans-perineal biopsy and multi-parametric MRI to the diagnostic pathway.

B. Challacombe
Department of Urology, Guy's and St Thomas
NHS Foundation Trust, Great Maze Pond, London SE1 9RT, UK
e-mail: benchallacombe@doctors.org.uk

B. Challacombe, S. Bott (eds.), *Diagnostic Techniques in Urology*, 9
DOI 10.1007/978-1-4471-2766-6_2,
© Springer-Verlag London 2014

TRUS Biopsy

This biopsy usually occurs with the man lying on his left side with the knees drawn up to the chest. Local anaesthetic is injected into the peri-prostatic tissues and occasionally sedation or light general anaesthetic can be used. Ten or twelve core samples are taken (5 or 6 from each side). Occasionally more samples are taken if the prostate gland is particularly large. Side effects of this technique include rectal and urethral bleeding and haematospermia. An increasing issue is that of post biopsy urinary infection which can lead to fulminant sepsis in rare cases. Recent overseas travel and antibiotic use are also independent risk factors for severe infection after prostate biopsy, with a 2.7-fold and fourfold increase in risk, respectively [1]. When infections do occur, they are usually caused by multidrug-resistant *E. coli*; accordingly, additional care—such as delay before biopsy, different antibiotic prophylaxis (such as meropenem) or transperineal biopsy—should be considered in these cases. Other rarer side effects include bleeding causing clot retention, worsening lower urinary tract symptoms and urinary retention, and temporary erectile dysfunction.

TRUS-guided biopsy has several advantages over the transperineal approach for sampling the prostate, which include taking less time to perform, costing less, requiring only readily available equipment and being highly reproducible and easy to teach. Some men have had several TRUS biopsies for a persistently rising PSA when previous biopsies have shown no cancer.

Trans-perineal Biopsy

Trans-perineal biopsy involves passing needles into the prostate directly through the perineal skin thus avoiding piercing the rectum. The ultrasound probe to guide the sampling still occurs trans rectally. This technique usually involves a general or spinal anaesthetic but can occasionally be performed with sedation. It is easier to sample all of the prostate and many more cores can be taken (usually 24–36) with some centres mapping the entire prostate with 60–90 cores [2, 3].

Transperineal prostate biopsy is at present making a comeback after decades of being an underused alternative to TRUS biopsy. Factors driving this change include possible improved cancer detection rates, improved sampling of the anteroapical regions of the prostate, a reduced risk of false negative results and a reduced risk of underestimating disease volume and grade. For transperineal biopsy, equipment is more expensive and is currently less freely available than that required for the TRUS approach. Indeed, better probes, disposable grids and—if fusing images with MRI—a high specification MRI machine is required. The increasing incidence of antimicrobial resistance and patients with diabetes mellitus who are at high risk of sepsis also favours transperineal biopsy as a sterile alternative to standard TRUS-guided biopsy. Factors limiting its use include increased time, training and financial constraints as well as the need for high-grade anaesthesia. Furthermore, the necessary equipment for transperineal biopsy is not widely available.

Side effects include urethral bleeding and haematospermia but not rectal bleeding, worsening lower urinary tract symptoms, urinary retention and temporary erectile dysfunction. Urinary infection is much rarer with this technique and urinary sepsis almost never seen. Whether transperineal biopsy of the prostate has a role as an initial investigation or should be reserved only for patients with previous negative transrectal biopsies remains under debate. The change of malignant seeding for either TRUS or trans-perineal biopsy is thought to be very minimal.

MRI

MRI technology has an increasing role in improving the yield of current prostate biopsy protocols [4]. As a method of staging biopsy proven prostate cancer an MRI is recommended for all intermediate and high risk disease to give staging both around the prostate (T staging) and regionally for both lymphadenopathy and metastases (N, M staging). To reduce biopsy artefact, MRI should ideally be performed at least 4–6 weeks after prostate biopsy, at a magnetic strength of least 1.5 T. Despite this much post-biopsy artefact is seen from haemorrhage and inflammation and can persist for up to 6 months so MRI is increasingly being used prior to biopsy to give a clearer set of images. Multiparametric MRI using gadolinium contrast and diffusion weighting enables the prostate to be evaluated in a number of differing series to improve sensitivity and specificity. It is currently often diffi-cult to access in busy hospitals, costly and can be claustropho-bic to the patient (see Chap. 4 for more on prostate MRI).

MRI Guided Biopsy

With the increasing placement of MRI prior to the prostate biopsy in the diagnostic pathway for suspected prostate can-cer this has led to a knock-on effect. Often abnormal lesions are detected on MRI within the prostate which are suspicious for prostate cancer permitting targeting of these areas at sub-sequent biopsy.

There are currently two methods for targeting these areas. In the first method, the urologist makes a mental note of the location of a target lesion found on prebiopsy MRI scan and tries to sample it with a TRUS-guided or transperi-neal approach, in a process known as cognitive-directed biopsy. The other method, known as fusion-guided MRI biopsies, requires the MRI scans are to be computerized and assimilated together with real-time ultrasonography guid-ance—usually TRUS—during the actual biopsy procedure to enable improved targeting [5, 6]. Whichever method is used to guide the needles, most feel that a trans-perineal biopsy route under general anaesthetic improves accuracy and control.

Rising PSA Despite Previous Negative TRUS Biopsy

This is a relatively common and worrying situation for both the patient and the physician. Clues can be sought from a history of urinary infection or prostatitis causing the PSA to be elevated or from PSA density and free/total ration (see Chap. 1) but often another biopsy is contemplated. In the past many men had multiple sets of TRUS biopsies for a persistently rising PSA despite previous negative TRUS biopsies. These generally have reported low cancer detection rates of 10–23 % in the second set of TRUS-guided biopsies and 5–14 % for the third set [7]. Growing evidence supports the use of transperineal biopsy in men at high risk of developing prostate cancer who have prior negative TRUS-guided biopsy results, which is a particular issue for men with larger prostates or an anterior or apical zone tumour. In patients with two or more prior negative TRUS-guided biopsies, prostate cancer detection rates by transperineal template-guided biopsy range from 50 to 68 %. In a study of 373 patients, transperineal template-guided biopsy detected prostate cancer in 41.7 % of men with two and 34.4 % of men with three or more prior negative transrectal biopsies. Such detection rates are encouraging in view of the relatively low cancer detection rates achieved with repeated TRUS-guided biopsies.

Currently the NIH and the UK National Institute for Clinical Excellence (NICE) recommends that transperineal biopsy can be indicated for patients with suspected prostate cancer who have had a negative or inconclusive TRUS-guided biopsy. As described above a multi-parametric MRI scan prior to a secondary biopsy may also provide valuable information and permit potential targeting of suspicious lesions.

Suggested Diagnostic Pathway: prior to this series.

Elevated PSA/Abnormal DRE → Multi-parametric MRI → Trans-perineal biopsy → Treatment or discharge.

> Success does not consist of never making mistakes but in never making the same one a second time.
>
> George Bernard Shaw

References

1. Patel U, et al. Infection after transrectal ultrasonography-guided prostate biopsy: increased relative risks after recent international travel or antibiotic use. BJU Int. 2012;109(12):1781–5.
2. Bott SR, et al. Extensive transperineal template biopsies of prostate: modified technique and results. Urology. 2006;68:1037–41.
3. Vyas L, et al. Indications, results and safety profile of transperineal sector biopsies of the prostate: a single centre experience of 634 cases. BJU Int. 2014;114(1):32–7.
4. Raz O, Haider M, Trachtenberg J, Leibovici D, Lawrentschuk N. MRI for men undergoing active surveillance or with rising PSA and negative biopsies. Nat Rev Urol. 2010;7(10):543–51.
5. Pinto PA, et al. Magnetic resonance imaging/ultrasound fusion guided prostate biopsy improves cancer detection following transrectal ultrasound biopsy and correlates with multiparametric magnetic resonance imaging. J Urol. 2011;186(4):1281–5.
6. Hadaschik BA, et al. A novel stereotactic prostate biopsy system integrating pre-interventional magnetic resonance imaging and live ultrasound fusion. J Urol. 2011;186(6):2214–20.
7. Roehl KA, Antenor JA, Catalona WJ. Serial biopsy results in prostate cancer screening study. J Urol. 2002;167:2435–9.

Chapter 3
Abnormal Digital Rectal Examination

James Duthie, Helen Freeborn, and Declan G. Murphy

Introduction

Despite advances in imaging techniques, and evaluation of blood and urine markers, the digital rectal examination (DRE) remains a cornerstone of the urological assessment. Barriers to effective DRE remain embarrassment (of both the patient and the clinician), lack of thorough assessment (the "nominal" examination), and a lack of experience causes misinterpretation of results. An abnormal DRE almost always requires further investigation.

J. Duthie • H. Freeborn • D.G. Murphy (✉)
Division of Cancer Surgery, Peter MacCallum Cancer Centre,
University of Melbourne, East Melbourne, VIC 3002, Australia
e-mail: declan.murphy@petermac.org

B. Challacombe, S. Bott (eds.), *Diagnostic Techniques in Urology*, 15
DOI 10.1007/978-1-4471-2766-6_3,
© Springer-Verlag London 2014

From a urological point of view, DRE is indicated most commonly due to lower urinary tract symptoms (LUTS), haematuria, infertility, or as part of prostate cancer screening in association with a PSA test. With the advent of PSA testing, a DRE test to help confirm a prostatic primary in a symptomatic man with newly discovered metastatic cancer is now thankfully rare.

Examination

The patient is consented, and then allowed to disrobe from the waist down in private. The DRE may be performed with the patient either in the left lateral position with hips and knees flexed, or upright, bending at the waist with elbows on the examination table. A sheet is used until the last possible moment to preserve dignity (Fig. 3.1).

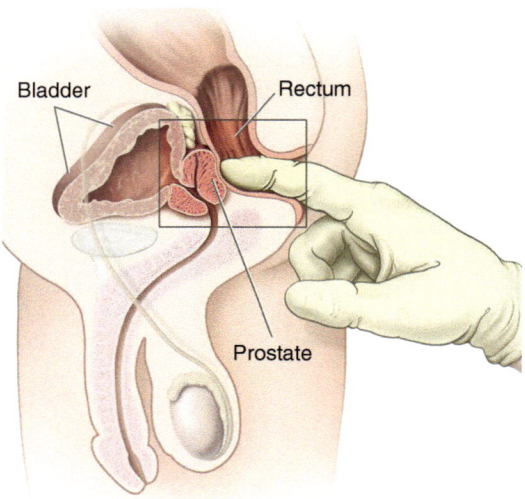

FIGURE 3.1 Digital rectal examination of the prostate (Image courtesy of the National Cancer Institute http://www.cancer.gov/dictionary?cdrid=45668)

As with all medical examination, performing the DRE provides a great deal of information to the examiner. With the buttocks parted, anal tags, haemorrhoids, anal fissures or fistulae may be identified. A severely excoriated or inflamed anus may be too tender to allow examination. In the upright position, the lubricated index finger of the prone dominant hand is gently inserted into the anus. In the left lateral position the table is raised to a comfortable height for the examiner, and the right index finger is inserted into the anus. The examiner then twists their arm to allow the pad of the finger to rest on the prostate in the anterior aspect of the rectum and some examiners may choose to kneel or crouch so that their finger is horizontal to the floor.

Anal tone is noted, and normal sensation can be confirmed with the patient if relevant. A circumferential examination of the rectum is essential as missing an easily palpable mucosal lesion is indefensible. DRE may be more difficult in the obese patient, the man with restricted lower limb movement, or when the examiner has short fingers.

Prostate

The prostate is identified anteriorly, and an assessment of the surface from apex to base is made. Relevant information includes both symptoms and signs:

A tender prostate is consistent with prostatitis, and discretion is used with further examination to avoid causing unnecessary patient discomfort. Objectively, size, consistency, and nodularity are relevant features.

Size

The normal prostate is approximately 20 cc in volume, with distinct left and right lobes and central sulcus palpable. This distinction maybe lost with significant BPH. Although increasing prostate volume is only poorly related to increasing LUTS, size estimation is important in directing further management. For example, 5-α reductase inhibitors are more effective with larger prostates. A small prostate in the context of a raised PSA level increases the suspicion of malignancy, as there is little benign prostatic hyperplasia (BPH) to explain the elevation. It is important to remember that asymptomatic prostatic enlargement is not an indication for treatment.

Consistency

The normal prostate is firm but rubbery in texture, commonly compared to the consistency of a flexed thenar eminence. BPH tissue is similarly yielding, and differs from the hard consistency of malignancy.

In acute prostatitis the prostate may have a "boggy" consistency, and is usually exquisitely tender. Chronic infection may lead to an indurated gland. Abscesses may be difficult to palpate, and imaging is more useful for confirmation. A cystic swelling in the midline may be the result of a prostate utricle cyst or obstructed ejaculatory ducts in the infertile male. Rarely in the developed world, granulomas due to tuberculosis may be palpated.

Nodularity

Both cancer and benign tissue may be nodular, and it should be remembered that a palpable nodule has an approximately 60 % chance of yielding malignant tissue on needle biopsy [3]. If in doubt, a biopsy to rule out carcinoma should be strongly considered. The location and estimated size of nodules must be recorded for future reference.

Seminal Vesicles

The seminal vesicles (SV) are impalpable unless pathology is present. Malignant infiltration will cause hardening of the

SV, synonymous with T3b prostate cancer but also encountered in locally advanced bladder cancer. The SV may be tense and dilated in ejaculatory duct obstruction.

Further Investigations

Blood and urine investigations, imaging, and biopsy are performed as appropriate according to DRE findings.

A tender prostate, particularly in the setting of fever and LUTS supports a diagnosis of acute prostatitis and a full blood count, and urinalysis, culture and sensitivities are indicated. Acute bacterial prostatitis is almost always due to Gram negative sepsis, and should therefore be treated aggressively and expeditiously. Antibiotic therapy should never be delayed while a microbe is isolated. Unusually, an abscess may form following bacterial prostatitis, giving ongoing fevers and LUTS past the expected 48–72 h course. Imaging with either trans-rectal ultrasound or MRI will confirm the diagnosis. For diagnosis of chronic prostatitis a 2- or 4-glass Meares-Stamey test may be considered.

If the indication for DRE is haematuria, imaging of the renal tract is mandatory, as is cystoscopy with a few exceptions. Urine cytology, or use of other urine biomarkers is not universally agreed upon, but may be useful. Ultrasound has been demonstrated to be acceptable for patients at low risk of urothelial malignancy, while 3-phase CT is preferred for those at high risk.

If the indication for DRE is LUTS, the usual adjuncts of urinary flow rate, urinalysis, symptom score assessment, PSA, and renal tract ultrasound where indicated are performed. Although uncommonly a cause of LUTS, prostate cancer must be ruled out before BPH may be assumed. A flow rate suspicious for urethral stricture should be followed by cysto-urethroscopy, and urethrogram if anything more than the simplest of strictures is encountered.

As discussed above, a PSA is always performed for prostate cancer screening, and may be a trigger for biopsy to rule out prostate cancer even in the context of a normal DRE.

If a suspicious nodule, or area of induration is palpated, a biopsy is indicated in any man who would benefit from management of a potential prostate cancer. In the context of newly discovered metastatic disease and a very high PSA (>100 ng/ml), a definitely malignant-feeling prostate may obviate the need for biopsy before starting urgent hormone manipulation. In the rare patient at risk of prostatic tuberculosis, daily early morning urine should be collected for acid-fast bacilli testing, culture and sensitivity, and perhaps PCR. If not already performed, an erect chest x-ray is mandatory.

Palpable, hardened SV raise suspicion for malignancy, and usually a PSA, renal tract imaging, and perhaps cystoscopy are indicated to rule out prostatic and urothelial malignancy. In the context of infertility, dilated SV or a palpable midline cyst require imaging with either TRUS or MRI. Identifiable ejaculatory duct obstruction may be treatable with transurethral resection. Vasogram is rarely of material benefit in these cases, and is rarely employed.

The Value of DRE in Prostate Cancer Diagnosis

Prior to the use of PSA for the detection of prostate cancer, clinicians relied solely on the DRE. The DRE as a screening tool for prostate cancer has a sensitivity ranging from 59 to 67 % with reported specificity ranging from 18 to 99 % [3]. The reproducibility of a DRE in experienced clinicians has best been described as fair [7]. When used alone DRE does miss a substantial number of the cancers that were subsequently detected by prostate biopsies done for serum PSA elevations or for transrectal ultrasound (TRUS) abnormalities [4], and is therefore not adequate for excluding prostate cancer. The DRE does, however, detect some prostate cancers that are missed by PSA screening [2, 6] as DRE and PSA do not always detect the same cancers [5]. A suspicious DRE is therefore an indication for prostate biopsy in men who would be candidates for treatment.

When DRE is used in conjunction with PSA, the detection rate for prostate cancer is higher than with PSA or DRE alone [1], hence the combination is recommended by many authorities for screening.

References

1. Catalona W, Smith D, Ratliff T, Dodds K, Coplen D, Yuan J, Petros J, Andriole G. Measurement of prostate- specific antigen in serum as a screening test for prostate cancer. New Engl J Med. 1991;324:1156–61.
2. Godley P. Prostate cancer screening: promise and peril—a review. Cancer Detect Prev. 1999;23:316–24.
3. Mistry K, Cable G. Meta-analysis of prostate-specific antigen and digital rectal examination as screening tests for prostate carcinoma. J Am Board Fam Med. 2003;16(2):95–101.
4. Ng T, Vasilareas D, Mitterdorfer A, Maher P, Lalak A. Prostate cancer detection with digital rectal examination, prostate-specific antigen, transrectal ultrasonography and biopsy in clinical urological practice. Brit J Urol Int. 2005;95(4):545–8.
5. Okotie O, Roehl K, Han M, Loeb S, Gashti S, Catalona W. Characteristics of prostate cancer detected by digital rectal examination only. Urology. 2007;70(6):1117–20.
6. Schroder F, van der Maas P, Beemsterboer P, Kruger A, Hoedemaeker R, Rietbergen J, Kranse R. Evaluation of the digital rectal examination as a screening test for prostate cancer. Rotterdam section of the European Randomized Study of Screening for Prostate Cancer. J Natl Cancer I. 1998;90(23): 1817–23.
7. Smith D, Catalona W. Interexaminer variability of digital rectal examination in detecting prostate cancer. Urology. 1995;45(1): 70–4.

Chapter 4
Imaging of Prostate Specific Symptoms

Anisha Patel, Farzana Rahman, and Uday Patel

Radiological Investigation of the Man with an Elevated PSA or Suspected Prostate Cancer

There is a pressing need to try and identify the men with a raised PSA who harbour a significant cancer; both to identify men with potentially life threatening prostate cancer and also to avoid unnecessary prostate biopsies in those without significant disease. Radiological techniques are rapidly evolving in this area, though much of the data is currently immature

A. Patel, FRCR • F. Rahman, FRCR
Department of Radiology, St George's Hospital,
Blackshaw Road, London, UK

U. Patel (✉)
Department of Radiology, St George's Hospital and Medical
School, Blackshaw Road, London, SW 17 0QT, UK
e-mail: uday.patel@stgeorges.nhs.uk

B. Challacombe, S. Bott (eds.), *Diagnostic Techniques in Urology*,   23
DOI 10.1007/978-1-4471-2766-6_4,
© Springer-Verlag London 2014

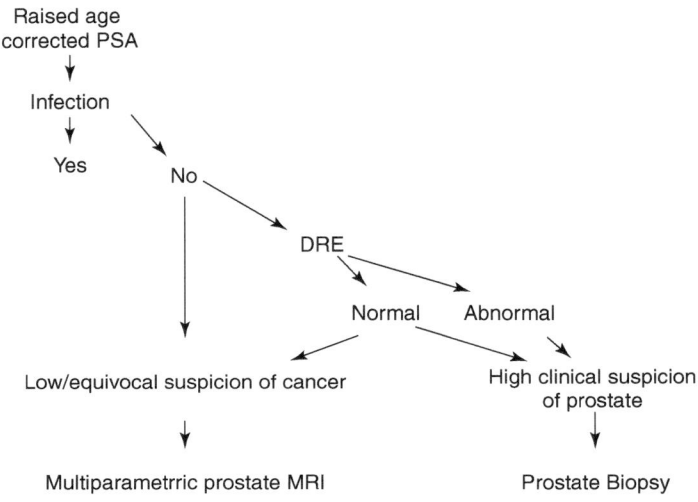

Transrectal Ultrasound (TRUS)

TRUS has a limited diagnostic accuracy, as most cancers, especially low volume or early tumours are either invisible on US or can not be differentiated from background BPH. The PPV of TRUS is said to be between 17 and 54 % and is dependent on PSA value (1) A 7-5-9 MHz end firing, or biplane transrectal probe is used. The whole gland is inspected in the transverse and longitudinal plane. Particular attention is paid to the 'blind zones' during prostate biopsy, i.e. regions often at the edge of the field of view; such as the posterolateral margins (or anterior horns), the base, apex and anterior gland. The normal prostate is symmetrical and homogeneous. Any nodular or diffuse echotexture changes should be treated as suspicious, especially those of increased vascularity or capsular irregularity. Colour Doppler ultrasound, elastography or contrast enhanced TRUS can improve accuracy, but only by a further 10 %. Tumour is more likely to be of increased vascularity or relative 'hardness' on elastography.

Multiparametric Magnetic Resonance Imaging of the Prostate Gland (mpMRI)

MRI in prostate cancer has shown promise for pre-biopsy, post PSA risk stratification. Initial data suggest a NPV of 95 %, and sensitively and specificity of around 80 %, but the positive predicative value may be as low as 40 %; and this is using a standardized reporting template and the best quality multiparametric MRI protocols. Multiparametric implies, that as well as basic anatomic imaging (using T2 weighted scans) there are additional 'physiological' studies. Ideally there should be two further sequences, most commonly these are diffusion weighted sequences (DWI with ADC maps) and dynamic contrast enhanced series. Some centers use spectroscopy as well.

Focused thin slice axial, coronal and sagittal T2, diffusion weighted and dynamic contrast enhanced studies focused on the prostate gland are imperative for maximal diagnostic accuracy. Tumours are depicted as low T2 signal foci, and as areas of increased cellularity (high signal intensity on the DWI series) or restricted diffusion (low signal intensity on the ADC maps) and augmented vascularity (with early avid vascular blush and rapid washout). An abnormal focus on all sequences is highly likely to be high grade tumour regardless of volume, or intermediate grade and large volume (the definition of a 'high volume' is has not been clearly defined, but thought to be a tumour of diameter ≥ 1 cm). Small volume/or low grade multifocal tumours are likely to be missed or lie in the intermediate category. A 5-point grading system can be used to quantify diagnostic certainty. Grades 1–2 denote certain or highly likely benign focus, grade 3 implies that a cancer can not be confirmed or excluded, whilst grades 4 and 5 imply a high likelihood or near certainty of the presence of tumour. The same scoring can be used for anterior grade tumours, but the accuracy is less than the figures given above. However, many glands fall in the grade 3 category as background inflammation and/or BPH will display low level changes in any, sometimes all, MRI sequences.

Radiological Investigation of Prostatitis (or Chronic Pelvic Pain)

Prostatitis can be classified as:

- Catergory I: Acute bacterial prostatitis (ABP)
- Catergory II: Chronic bacterial prostatitis (CBP)
- Catergory III: Chronic prostatitis and chronic pelvic pain syndrome (divided into inflammatory IIIa and non inflammatory causes IIIb)
- Catergory IV: Asymptomatic inflammatory prostatitis

Only a small number of men with prostatitis have true bacterial infection. The majority are classified as category III when symptomatic or category IV if asymptomatic. In clinical practice most are in the third category. Increasingly this symptom complex is considered under the broad heading of chronic pelvic pain syndrome. Most cases of clinically evident prostatitis do not require any specific radiological imaging.

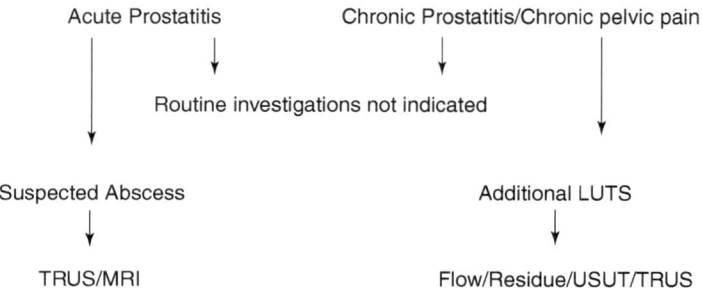

MRI

MRI is not used to routinely image prostatitis. However, it is important to be aware of the appearances of prostatitis on MRI in order to distinguish it from prostate cancer. Prostatitis may also co-exist with prostate malignancy; therefore it is important that it is identified so that prostate cancer is not upstaged. Prostate cancer typically appears as a discrete signal T2 focus in the peripheral zone, with increased cellularity and restricted diffusion on DWI MRI and is of increased, early phase vascularity on post contrast studies. In the central and transition zones, cancer is demonstrated as a homogenous low signal intensity area with poorly defined borders and difficult to distinguish form background BPH. Prostatitis may mimic prostate cancer and can also exhibit diffuse low T2 signal in the peripheral zone. It can be difficult to differentiate it from prostate cancer but a suggestive feature is a more diffuse striated low T2 signal intensity with inflammation, in contrast to the discrete focus seen with prostate carcinoma. Distinguishing features on DWI studies and spectroscopy have not yet been defined. The overlap in imaging features means that correlation with clinical symptoms is vital.

Transrectal Ultrasound

Acute prostatitis may manifest without any imaging findings but described features include increased gland vascularity which may either be diffuse or focal. The gland can be of generalised low echogenicity with loss of the normal anatomical boundaries, or contain focal echo-poor areas and have a thick walled capsule. An acute abscess will appear as a focal cystic area with a thick wall, and can be easily drained under TRUS guidance. Chronic prostatitis has non-specific imaging features which can include distension of the periprostatic veins, a dystrophic inner gland, periurethral calcification or hyperechoic thickening of the capsule. In contrast, granulomatous prostatitis has distinct ultrasound features, presenting as a bulging nodule of mixed echogenicity. The capsule and the periprostatic fat planes will be intact, unlike the findings with prostate carcinoma.

Radiological Investigation of the Man with Haematospermia or Suspected Obstructive Infertility

An isolated episode of haematospermia is common and unlikely to require radiological investigation. Repeated episodes may benefit from detailed assessment. The common benign causes of haematospermia can be broadly divided into congenital, inflammatory or obstructive causes. Bleeding into congenital cysts in the seminal vesicles/ejaculatory ducts or into Müllerian duct remnants may be associated with haematospermia. Ejaculatory duct calculi or prostatitis may also result in haematospermia. Malignancy, either of the prostate gland or the seminal vesicles, is a very rare cause. Extra-testicular obstructive infertility may be due to congenital or acquired absence or obstruction of the ejaculatory ducts or seminal vesicles resulting in a low or absent sperm count. TRUS is the modality of choice for the radiological investigation of either of these two symptom complexes. MRI does not generally contribute any further information.

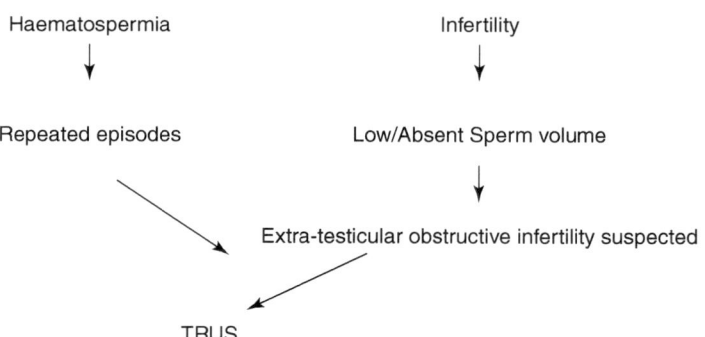

TRUS and MRI

Blood products or sperm in the duct or seminal vesicles may be seen as an echogenic layer. On MRI, blood products have a unique signature, being of high T1 signal, and low T2 signal. Stone or calcification in the ejaculatory ducts are seen as reflective discrete or diffuse structures within the lumen, and easily identified on TRUS. In comparison, small calculi are very difficult to see on MRI, as they do not have any signal. The upstream duct and seminal vesicle may be dilated. The normal ejaculatory duct has no measurable lumen. If the duct lumen is visualised than it is dilated. In comparison the lumen of the vesicles is normally visualised, and apparent dilatation may be due physiological distension. If in doubt, the scan should be repeated after ejaculation, in which case physiological distension will improve. Cystic anomalies may be associated with haematospermia or obstruction. Utricle cysts cannot be reliably differentiated from remnant cysts on TRUS, but the latter are said to be larger and more likely to extend above the gland.

Of other radiological investigations, scrotal ultrasound is useful for confirming testicular size. Seminal vesiculography, undertaken as an open procedure or under transrectal ultrasoundguidance, can help confirm the level of ejaculatory duct obstruction.

Radiological Staging of Prostate Cancer

The major challenge with prostate cancer is its wide variety, ranging from asymptomatic and clinically insignificant disease to rapidly progressive systemic malignancy. Imaging can help stage prostate cancer for risk stratification and to assist treatment planning.

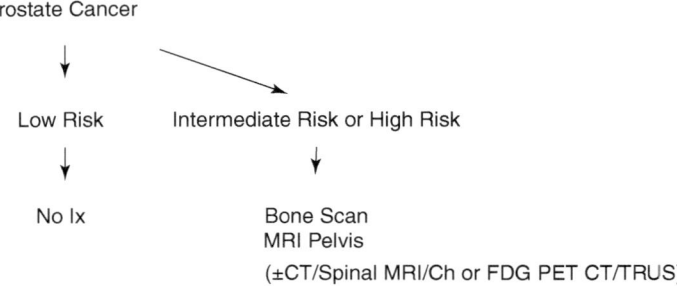

Prostate Cancer

Low Risk   Intermediate Risk or High Risk

No Ix   Bone Scan
                        MRI Pelvis
                        (±CT/Spinal MRI/Ch or FDG PET CT/TRUS)

Bone Scan

Bone scintigraphy uses a radioactive isotope attached to a molecule that accumulates in areas of increased bone turnover, thus it has a high sensitivity but low specificity. Essentially any area of osteoblastosis will light up, e.g. fractures, inflammation and benign osteoblastic process such as Paget's disease. Other modalities, even the relatively insensitive plain radiograph, may be later required to better delineate some lesions detected on bone scan. Another limitation is that a bone scan does not provide information on bony architecture, and again plain radiographs, MRI or CT may be used, e.g. for evaluation extra-osseous involvement and to exclude cord compression in those with spinal metastasis and neural symptoms.

Clinical risk status can be used to determine the necessity for screening bone scans. Those with low grade disease and PSA < 10 ng/ml. have a very low probability of occult bone metastasis, such that false positive bone findings such as rib fractures etc. are more likely.

Magnetic Resonance Imaging (MRI)

MRI of the prostate and pelvis is the best imaging modality for demonstrating intra-prostatic tumour volume and extra-capsular disease. CT and MRI are about equivalent for the evaluation of nodal spread. Spinal MRI is useful has a higher specificity than bone scan for metastasis, but is used for problem solving and is the only modality that will confirm suspected spinal cord compression/invasion.

Focused thin slice axial, coronal and sagittal T2 studies of the prostate are used for assessing zonal anatomy, the prostate capsule and seminal vesicle (SV) invasion. Axial T1 weighted images of the pelvis up to the level of the aortic bifurcation will detect nodal metastases. Additional studies, such as diffusion weighted MRI and post contrast dynamic enhanced series help assessment of intra-glandular tumour volume, and assist local staging.

The zonal anatomy of the prostate and the seminal vesicles are optimally demonstrated on the T2 sequence. The normal peripheral zone has homogenous high T2 signal that can be equal to that of the surrounding fat. The central zone is low signal on T2, as is the fibromuscular stroma. The transition zone is of intermediate to low T2 signal. The prostatic capsule is a thin (<1 mm) low signal rim circumscribing the prostatic margin, although it is deficient at the apex and at the fibro-muscular stroma anteriorly. Carcinoma typically appears as low T2 against the normal background high signal peripheral zone. Carcinoma may be masked in the normally low signal central gland or if the peripheral zone is of heterogeneous signal intensity. Thus, a normal gland appearance does not exclude prostate cancer. Conversely, low T2 signal in the peripheral zone is not specific for prostate cancer; other causes include haemorrhage, prostatitis, dystrophic changes secondary to radiation or hormone deprivation therapy. Post biopsy haemorrhage can be mistaken for tumour and staging MRI should be delayed for at least 3 months after prostate biopsy, although sometimes such artifact can persist for many months. On the diffusion studies, tumour is seen as areas of high signal signifying increased cellularity and of low signal on the ADC maps, because of restricted diffusion. Tumours are more vascular than normal prostate tissue and so enhance with contrast with prompt washout.

MRI features most specific for ECE are obliteration of the rectoprostatic angle, asymmetry of the NVBs and irregularity or bulging of the capsule. Early tumour extension into the periprostatic fat causes loss of the normal fat plane separating the prostate and rectum posteriorly. In combination the findings of loss of recto-prostatic angle (RPA) and asymmetry of NVBs has a high specificity (up to 95 %) for early ECE, although sensitivity remains limited (<50 %).

The seminal vesicles are normally of high T2 signal due to their fluid content. Asymmetry is seen with tumour invasion. Other signs are low T2 signal and loss of the fat plane between the prostate and the SV. A high specificity (88 %) but low sensitivity (22 %) has been reported for SVI on MRI. Benign causes of low signal or asymmetry of the seminal vesicles include post-biopsy haemorrhage, chronic inflammation, radiation response and amyloidosis. Bladder invasion is suggested by loss of the fat plane between the prostate base and the bladder anteriorly, and disruption of the normal low signal of the muscular bladder wall. Extension into the rectum is reflected by loss of the fat plane between the prostate and rectum. Frank invasion will cause interruption of the normal signal intensity of the anterior rectal wall. The absolute indications for MRI use have yet to be universally agreed, MRI may have a role in the pre-biopsy setting to decide whether to biopsy the prostate in a man with a raised PSA and where to target the biopsy needles. MRI also has a role in the post biopsy setting in men with intermediate and high risk disease to assess for extra capsular extension (accepting there may be biopsy artifact for 3–6 months), nodal disease and pelvic boney metastases.

Computed Tomography (CT)

The primary role of CT in prostate cancer imaging is in the detection of distant disease.

The accuracy of CT in detecting pelvic and retroperitoneal nodal metastases is variable but sensitivities of up to 78 % and specificity of 97 % have been quoted (A) [11]. The primary CT sign for positive nodal disease is size. A short axis diameter of ≥1 cm being considered abnormal for para-aortic nodes, ≥9 mm for common iliac nodes and ≥8 mm for internal iliac and obturator nodes. Secondary signs of metastatic nodal disease is a rounded appearance of the node, an absence of fat in the centre or hilum or enhancement with intravenous contrast. Microscopic nodal metastases cannot be detected by either CT or MRI. False positive findings result when nodal enlargement occurs secondary to a benign etiology.

Gross local disease extension may be detectable on CT, for example extracapsular extension may be suggested if there is obliteration of the periprostatic fat plane. Seminal vesicle enlargement and asymmetry may indicate locally invasive disease, as may thickening and irregularity of the wall of the bladder or rectum.

Distant spread in the form of bone, liver and lung metastases are uncommon but may also be detected. CT can help differentiate malignant from benign causes of increased uptake on bone scan. CT may sometimes be used to better delineate the architecture of a bone deposit, any related complication and monitor disease response, although CT changes may lag behind therapeutic response.

Other Radiological Modalities Used for Prostate Cancer Staging

Transrectal Ultrasound (TRUS)

TRUS has limited staging accuracy. The accuracy can be boosted by adjunct techniques such as colour Doppler US, contrast enhanced US or elastography but only marginally. It does have a role in problem solving, and occasionally for guiding seminal vesicle biopsy, or deep anterior gland biopsy, in the man with borderline seminal vesicle changes or a suspected undersampled anterior gland tumour on other staging modalities. Unlike MRI post biopsy artifact is not an issue.

The normal prostate gland is symmetrical and homogeneous. Any nodular or diffuse echotexture changes should be treated as suspicious, especially those of increased vascularity or capsular irregularity. Extracapsular extension is be suggested by irregularity, bulging or discontinuity of the capsule adjacent to the hypoechoic lesion. Seminal vesicle extension may be seen as extension of the hypoechoic lesion into the usually fluid filled seminal vesicles, or be suspected if there is obvious asymmetry of the vesicles. Local nodes are seldom if ever seen, but more extensive local invasion, e.g. the rectal wall, or bladder may be recognized.

PET-CT

PET- CT has a role in problem solving. Choline PET-CT is useful for soft tissue disease, as well as bone disease. But the accuracy has been reported to be about 70 % and performance is poor for nodes < 1 cm in diameter. FDG PET has a very high accuracy for bone disease, and can be used for evaluation of equivocal bone scan findings. The role of spinal MRI has already been discussed above.

Radiological Investigation of the Man with LUTS

The prostate gland undergoes hyperplasia beginning in the fourth decade, and after the fifth decade, 50 % of men will have some degree of BPH. Enlargement is not uniform. The transition zone is preferentially affected, with the peripheral and central zones relatively spared. Growth of the stromal and glandular elements occur in a diffuse or focal manner, the latter in the form of discrete adenomas. However the degree of BPH does not correlate with the severity or nature of the lower urinary tract symptoms. Minimal enlargement may be markedly obstructive, yet very large glands may result in minimal lower urinary tract symptoms (LUTS).

The management of LUTS is primarily guided by subjective measurements of symptom severity. Radiological investigations are not routinely necessary. However, there is a sub-group in whom further investigation may help e.g. the man with LUTS and reduced renal function or infection. Prostate size may also help guide treatment. Glands < 40 ml are better managed by alpha blockers, while those > 40 ml may be selected for 5 alpha reductase agents. Size may also help surgical planning. Mildly enlarged glands (<30 ml) may be suitable for bladder neck incision rather than TURP. Large glands (subjectively defined as those > 80 ml in volume - EAU) may be better treated by holmium laser enucleation (HoLEP) or rarely open prostatectomy rather than TURP; and the size of the 'median' lobe may also influence choice of treatment modality.

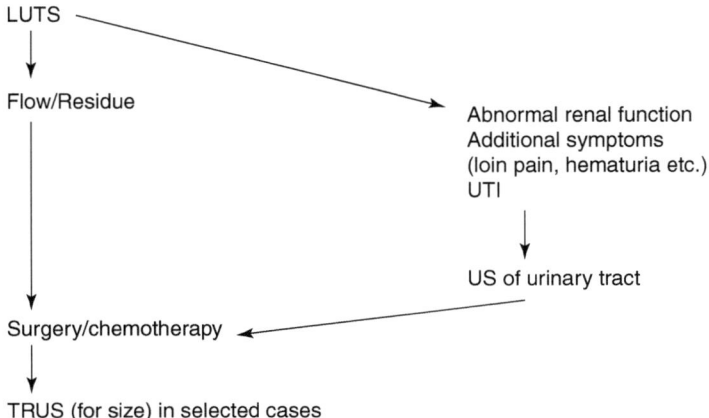

Urinary Tract Ultrasound

The upper tracts are preferentially investigated by ultrasound because of its safety, low cost, good renal mass evaluation and simultaneous assessment of the bladder. It should be reserved for cases with abnormal renal function and/or large post-void residual, specifically to look for hydronephrosis. Bladder wall thickness (normal < 3 mm) on ultrasound correlates with degree of outflow obstruction. In addition pre- and post-voiding bladder volume (formula : $H \times W \times L \times 0.52$) can be measured. Bladder stones should be excluded and if a significant diverticulum is seen, its position and its size before and after voiding should be measured, as it may act as a reservoir resulting in urinary frequency and post-voiding symptoms. Other significant findings including bladder, renal and urethral carcinoma have been reported to be detected in approximately 1 % of cases.

Transrectal Ultrasound of the Prostate Gland (TRUS)

TRUS is more accurate than DRE for prostate sizing, partly because it can account for any 'median' lobe enlargement. A number of formulae have been devised. The most convenient considers the prostate shape as akin to a prolate ellipsoid – length $\times$ height $\times$ width $\times \pi/6$ (or 0.52). An error margin of $\pm$ up to 20 % should be assumed, especially with larger glands. The most accurate measurement is by planimetry.

Typical TRUS findings of BPH are lobar asymmetry, an elevated bladder base and deviation of the urethra. The inner gland will be hypoechoic and heterogeneous, with compression of the peripheral zone, which consequently appears more hyperechoic. Discrete adenomas may be discernible and are usually well defined and of mixed reflectivity. The adenomas may demonstrate peripheral vascularity but should not have internal vascularity. They need to be differentiated from central gland tumours; these are usually uniformly hypoechoic with indistinct edges and some internal vascularity. Importantly, however enlarged the prostate may be, the capsule should remain intact. A breached capsule is seen with prostate cancer.

Other Investigations

More involved urinary tract investigations such as CT Urogram; and static or micturating cystography are not routinely recommended.

Further Reading

Radiological Investigation of the Man with an Elevated PSA or Suspected Prostate Cancer

1. Barentsz JO, Richenberg J, Clements R, Choyke P, Verma S, Villeirs G, Rouviere O, Logager V, Fütterer JJ. ESUR prostate MR guidelines 2012. Eur Radiol. 2012;22(4):746–57.
2. Dahm P, Dmochcowski R, editors. Evidence based urology. 2nd ed. Oxford: BMJ books/Wiley; 2010.
3. Heidenreich A, Bastian P.J, Bellmunt J, Bolla M, Joniau S, Mason MD, Matveev V, Mottet N, van der Kwast TH, Wiegel T, Zattoni F. Guidelines on prostate cancer. Available at http://www.uroweb.org/guidelines/online-guidelines/. Accessed 28 Aug 2013.
4. Portalez D, Mozer P, Cornud F, Renard-Penna R, Misrai V, Thoulouzan M, Malavaud B. Validation of the European Society of Urogenital Radiology scoring system for prostate cancer diagnosis on multiparametric magnetic resonance imaging in a cohort of repeat biopsy patients. Eur Urol. 2012;62(6):986–96.

Radiological Investigation of Prostatitis (or Chronic Pelvic Pain)

5. Fall M, Baranowski AP, Elneil S, Engeler D, Hughes J, Messelink EJ, Oberpenning F, de C. Williams AC. Guidelines on chronic pelvic pain. Uroweb 2011. Available at: http://www.uroweb.org/fileadmin/user_upload/Guidelines/Chronic%20Pelvic%20Pain.pdf Accessed 28 Aug 2013.
6. Patel U. The prostate and seminal vesicles. In: Allan PLP, Baxter GM, Weston MJ, editors. Clinical ultrasound. 3rd ed. Edinburgh: Churchill Livingstone; 2011.

7. Shukla-Dave A, Hricak H, Eberhardt SC, Olgac S, Muruganandham M, Scardino PT, Reuter VE, Koutcher JA, Zakian KL. Chronic prostatitis: MR imaging and 1H MR spectroscopic imaging findings–initial observations. Radiology. 2004;231(3):717–24.

Radiological Investigation of the Man with Haematospermia or Suspected Obstructive Infertility

8. Fisch H, Kang YM, Johnson CW, Goluboff ET. Ejaculatory duct obstruction. Curr Opin Urol. 2002;12(6):509–15.
9. Haematospermia. http://www.acr.org/Quality-Safety/Appropriateness-Criteria/Diagnostic/Urologic-Imaging. Accessed 28 Aug 2013.
10. Simpson Jr WL, Rausch DR. Imaging of male infertility: pictorial review. AJR Am J Roentgenol. 2009;192(6):98–107.

Radiological Staging of Prostate Cancer

11. Heidenreich A, Bastian P.J, Bellmunt J, Bolla M, Joniau S, Mason MD, Matveev V, Mottet N, van der Kwast T.H, Wiegel T, Zattoni F. Guidelines on prostate cancer. Available at http://www.uroweb.org/guidelines/online-guidelines/. Accessed 28 Aug 2013.
12. Husband JE, Reznek RH, editors. Imaging in oncology. 3rd ed. London: Informa Healthcare; 2013.
13. Prostate cancer diagnosis and treatment. Available at http://guidance.nice.org.uk/CG58/Guidance/pdf/English. Accessed 28 Aug 2013.

Radiological Investigation of the Man with LUTS

14. http://www.nice.org.uk/nicemedia/live/12984/48557/48557.pdf#page=9. Accessed 20 May 2013.
15. Oelke M, Bachmann A, Descazeaud A, Emberton M, Gravas S, Michel MC, N'dow J, Nordling J, de la Rosette JJ. EAU guidelines on the treatment and follow-up of non-neurogenic male lower urinary tract symptoms including benign prostatic obstruction. Eur Urol. 2013;64(1):118–40.

Chapter 5
Haematuria

Clarissa Martyn-Hemphill and Ben Challacombe

Haematuria refers to the presence of blood within the urine. This may be classified as 'visible' (previously termed 'gross' 'frank' or macroscopic) haematuria, which describes the pink to red discolouration of urine reported/observed, or non-visible (formerly microscopic or 'dipstick') haematuria. These classifications can be further sub-divided into 'symptomatic' presentations (*i.e.* associated pain/dysuria, frequency, urgency) or 'asymptomatic' episodes, which are often discovered incidentally on urinalysis.

Haematuria may be idiopathic or benign in origin. However, it remains the commonest presenting clinical feature of urological cancers (such as bladder and renal malignancies). Population-based screening studies have historically reported prevalence rates of asymptomatic, non-visible haematuria as approximately 2.5 % in the UK. This is not concordant with the number of urological malignancies subsequently diagnosed. In a previous large prospective cohort analysis,

C. Martyn-Hemphill
Department of Urology, Guy's and St. Thomas
NHS Foundation Trust, London, UK

B. Challacombe, MS FRCS (Urol) (✉)
Department of Urology, Guy's and St. Thomas NHS Foundation Trust, Great Maze Pond, London SE1 9RT, UK
e-mail: benchallacombe@doctors.org.uk

B. Challacombe, S. Bott (eds.), *Diagnostic Techniques in Urology*,   39
DOI 10.1007/978-1-4471-2766-6_5,
© Springer-Verlag London 2014

TABLE 5.1 Causes of haematuria

Urological	Nephrological	Spurious	Other

Malignancy
  Bladder (TCC, SCC)
  Kidney (RCC)
  Collecting system (TCC)
  Prostate
	Vasculitis
	
	Glomerulonephritides
	
	Polycystic kidney diease
	
	IgA nephropathy
		Food (beeturia)
		
		Drug use
		  Rifampicin
		  Nitrofurantoin
		  Doxorubicin
			Blood disorders
			  Sickle cell disease
			Exercise-induced
			
			Myoglobinuria

Calculi
  Renal
  Bladder
  Ureteric
		Menstruation (females)
		
		Sexual intercourse
			Intermittent Porphyria
			
			Post procedural e.g. catheterisation

Infection
  Cystitis
  Pyelonephritis
  Schistosomiasis (bilharzia)			

Trauma Benign prostatic hyperplasia Strictures Anatomical abnormalities Nutcracker Syndrome			

the overall prevalence rate of malignancy was 12.1 % of 4,020 patient referrals with haematuria (18.9 % visible and 4.8 % non-visible haematuria) [1]. Other studies have reported higher pick up rates with 35 % of visible and 19 % of cases of non-visible haematuria found to have a significant cause [2]. Although routine urinalysis screening in primary care is not currently recommended, further investigation is indicated in all new episodes of haematuria identified. Disease severity is not proportional to the number of episodes or severity of haematuria reported.

A systematic review by the National Institute of Health Research (NIHR HTA) in 2006 [3] demonstrated a paucity of evidence to support definitive investigations in the management of this common urological condition. This is due to the diversity of patient factors and extended spectrum of differential diagnoses (Table 5.1) derived from this clinical feature.

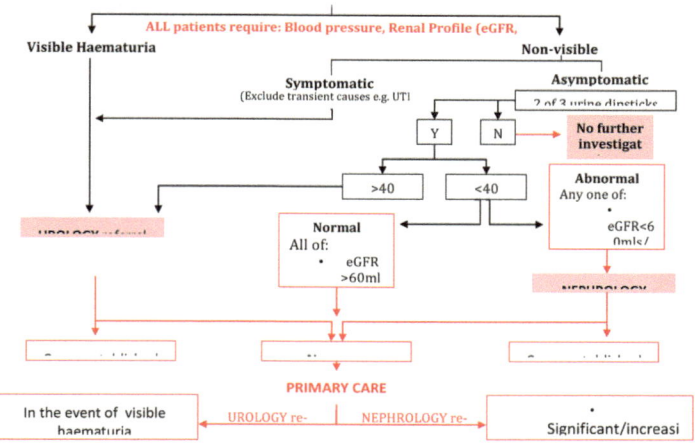

FIGURE 5.1 Decision algorithm for the investigation of haematuria (Adapted from proposed joint guidelines from the British Association of Urological Surgeons and the Renal Association)

However, these can be appropriately discriminated through use of the joint British Association of Urological Surgeons (BAUS) and Renal Association (RA) proposed diagnostic algorithm, as an adjunct to good clinical acumen (Fig. 5.1).

History

Haematuria may arise from any part of the urinary tract. The pattern of bleeding within the history may provide the clinician with information that helps focus the investigative approach to subsequent management. Once it has been established that the bleeding, if visible, is not originating from the patient's vagina or rectum, the clinician must assess duration and frequency of episodes; in addition to associated symptoms, or previous trauma, if applicable. Transient myoglobinuria for example, detected on urine dipstick as haematuria, should be suspected in patients with a history of recent excessive or strenuous exercise; a subsequently negative urinalysis result would obviate further investigation.

Visible haematuria noted at the onset of urination may be an indication of prostatic or urethral bleeding. Bladder or upper tract pathology can manifest with mid-stream or continuous haemorrhage. Terminal flow bleeding in the context of previous travel history may suggest schistosomiasis as the underlying cause for example. The presence of clots in the patient with haematuria, regardless of cause, can precipitate urinary clot retention in the male patient presenting acutely with no previous chronic obstructive cause identified. Similarly, the differential of 'clot colic' derived from occult renal malignancies, should be considered in the absence of upper tract stones in patients presenting with loin pain and haematuria. Likewise, a string of clot may indicate bleeding from the upper tracts whereas more rounded clots are likely to originate from in the bladder.

Visible or non-visible haematuria in the context of constitutional symptoms such as fever, dysuria and flank pain, suggest infection, requiring empirical antibiotic treatment. This should be confirmed with microscopy, culture and sensitivity results (MC + S) from a mid-stream urine sample (MSU). Urinary tract infections (UTI) almost universally represent a transient cause of haematuria that resolves with treatment. However, all patients over the age of 40 presenting with recurrent (greater than or equal to three episodes in 1 year) or persistent UTI warrant an referral to a urologist to rule out occult urological pathology.

Causes of haematuria are often identified within patients' past medical histories. Common co-morbidities such as diabetes, hypertension and sickle cell disease can constitute non-urological causes of nephropathic bleeding. This is often in association with proteinuria. All family histories should elucidate previous first-degree malignancies and potentially hereditary conditions such as von Hippel-Lindau syndrome (VHL), as well as autoimmune nephropathies.

A comprehensive drug history will not only identify allergy status, which may influence empiric antibiotic treatment choice in the event of infection, but also highlight transient causes of haematuria caused by medication.

The use of NSAIDS and/or cytotoxic drugs may precipitate haematuria secondary to interstitial renal damage. Note that although deranged clotting profiles derived from anti-coagulant and anti-platelet drugs may exacerbate haematuria, they should not be attributed as sole cause until underlying pathology has been excluded.

Tobacco smoking is the leading risk factor for bladder cancer, and is associated with 36 % of new cases per year in the UK [4]. It is important that each patient's smoking status is documented and clinicians are opportunistic about referring for smoking cessation if desired. Occupational exposure to carcinogens such as polycyclic aromatic hydrocarbons (PAHs) is thought to account for approximately 10 % of bladder cancers. Previous exposure should promote a low threshold for further investigation of patients in previous employments necessitating contact with dyes, paints and rubber manufacturing [5].

Assessment

Haematuria is quantified either by determining the number of red blood cells (RBC)/mm urine excreted (chamber count) or by analysis of urinary sediment. The indirect detection via urine dipstick measurement ($\geq 1 +$ blood) is an inexpensive and highly sensitive point of care test which can be confirmed on microscopy.

The presence of leucocytes and nitrites in the context of symptomatic non-visible haematuria signals infection requiring antibiotic treatment, as per local microbiology guidelines. Underlying tuberculosis should be considered in the event of sterile pyuria with concurrent, unexplained haematuria and relevant travel history or immunocompromised state. Proteinuria associated with haematuria and impaired renal function, is commonly associated with non-urological causes, such as diabetic, hypertensive or vascular nephropathies. The presence of casts on urinalysis is suggestive of underlying nephritides, related to glomerular damage. Clinical suspicion of any of the above warrants a referral to a renal physician. This must be accompanied by up to date blood pressure readings, renal profile (creatinine and eGFR) and full blood count. Additional urinary protein:creatinine and albumin:creatinine ratios (PCR/ACR) are also desirable to further evaluate renal function as per diagnostic algorithm (Fig. 5.1). A renal biopsy may be considered in these patients for investigation of potential underlying parenchymal disease.

All patients should undergo a full physical examination on initial presentation, to assess for systemic signs of illness. This should be undertaken in addition to a focussed urological assessment, which includes examination of the rectum, vagina and external genitalia. A PSA level is a mandatory accompaniment to all male referrals with associated LUTS or abnormal prostate on digital rectal exam but may be deferred if active infection is suspected.

Note that the clinician's priority in the initial management of acute visible haematuria is to identify and correct potential haemodynamic compromise related to hypovolaemia. Timely resuscitation with a systematic advanced life support (ALS) approach is essential. Some patients may require transfusion of blood products to restore normovolaemia and correct clotting abnormalities.

Imaging

Ultrasonography (USS) of the upper renal tract is the initial imaging modality of choice in the investigation of non-visible haematuria. It has replaced the routine use of excretory urography (IVU) as a quick, non-invasive, inexpensive outpatient tool with a high sensitivity for renal lesions. These include cysts, neoplasms, urolithiasis and evidence of obstructive masses causing hydronephrosis. USS also avoids the use of radiation, and negates adverse reactions such as anaphylaxis and renal impairment associated with use of intravenous contrast. This makes it safe for use during pregnancy and in chronic kidney disease. USS is of limited use however in the identification and differentiation of intra renal pelvic tumours and small parenchymal renal masses (*i.e.* less than 3 cm) which may require further imaging or radiologically-guided biopsies for definitive diagnosis.

CT urography (with contrast) is the modality of choice in the imaging of macroscopic haematuria [6]. Protocols vary according to the clinical history (e.g. recent abdominal trauma) and local guidelines. Generally, a non-contrast scan is performed initially to exclude a urinary tract stone. Contrast is then administered and a nephrographic phase scan is performed after approximately 60–90 min. This will highlight abnormalities in the renal parenchyma and help distinguish benign from malignant renal cysts. Finally, a pyleographic phase scan is undertaken 4 min after contrast injection to examine the renal collecting system, ureters and bladder. This will identify filling defects from transitional cell carcinoma, clot, gas etc.

Although essential for radiological staging of potentially invasive or metastatic disease, the choice of radiological imaging with CT or USS in the *initial* investigation of suspected lower urinary tract malignancy remains unclear.

Cystoscopy

Flexible cystoscopy enables direct visualisation of the lower urinary tract under local anaesthetic in the outpatient setting of the 'rapid-access' 'haematuria' clinic. This may detect mucosal lesions including carcinoma *in situ* (CIS) of the bladder, which may be missed using CT urography alone. Cystoscopy is an invasive, user-dependent procedure, which can be complicated by post-procedural bleeding and infection. If a suspicious lesion is visualised, patients are referred for a rigid cystoscopy, in which the transurethral resection of bladder tumours can provide histological diagnosis and grading.

The British and American Urological Societies recommend the investigation of haematuria with cystoscopy in all patients over 40 years old or in those with significant risk factors for bladder cancer of any age.

Cytology

Although relatively specific in the detection of high grade bladder tumours and CIS, cytology affords clinicians with a poor sensitivity rate and does not provide appropriate discriminant value as an investigative tool in patients with new-onset haematuria. The literature is concordant that this modality is not clinically or financially effective in this general diagnostic context.

Urinary Biomarkers e.g. NMP-22, BTA-Stat

There is growing interest in this area to provide a non-invasive diagnostic and surveillance alternative to cystoscopy to exclude urinary tract malignancies as the cause of haematuria. Initial results demonstrate inadequate specificity and poor positive predictive values in the investigation of patients with haematuria. At present, these do not replace cystoscopy in their rate of bladder tumour detection [7]. These are not currently recommended in routine practice, but may have an adjunctive role in the future, in combination with current modalities in the surveillance of patients with urological cancers.

Conclusion

- Visible haematuria is caused by underlying urological malignancy until proven otherwise.
- The severity of presentation will not necessarily correlate with that of the underlying cause.
- An appreciation of common causes of haematuria, their associated symptoms and knowledge of appropriate further investigations and referral pathways, will ensure timely investigation of this common urological presentation.
- All 'significant' new episodes require urgent investigation by a urologist as per the haematuria diagnostic algorithm (Fig. 5.1).

- Extensive investigation may not elicit the cause of haematuria in all patients.
- These individuals should be referred back to primary care for annual surveillance, with a low threshold for re-referral to a urologist or nephrologist, as appropriate, if symptoms recur in the interim.
- An awareness of evolving diagnostic techniques and the clinical implications of urinary cytology and biomarkers is advocated. Further research is needed to assess the comparative effectiveness of imaging modalities in the investigation of patients with new-onset visible or non-visible haematuria.

References

1. Edwards TJ, Dickinson AJ, Natale S, Gosling J, McGrath SJ. A prospective analysis of the diagnostic yield resulting from the attendance of 4020 patients at a protocol-driven haematuria clinic. BJU Int. 2006;97(2):301–5.
2. Khadra MH, Pickard RS, Charlton M, Powell PH, Neal DE. A prospective analysis of 1930 patients with haematuria to evaluate current diagnostic practice. J Urol. 2000;163:524–7.
3. Rodgers M, Nixon J, Hempel S, et al. Diagnostic tests and algorithms used in the investigation of haematuria: systematic reviews and economic evaluation. Health Technol Assess. 2006;10:iii–iv, xi–259.
4. Parkin DM. Tobacco-attributable cancer burden in the UK in 2010. Br J Cancer. 2011;105(S2):S6–13.
5. Kogevinas M, Mannetje A, Cordier S, Ranft U, González CA, Vineis P, Chang-Claude J, Lynge E, Wahrendorf J, Tzonou A. Occupation and bladder cancer among men in Western Europe. Cancer Causes Control. 2003;14(10):907–14.
6. Sadow CA, Silverman SG, O'Leary MP, Signorovitch JE. Bladder cancer detection with CT urography in an Academic Medical Center. Radiology. 2008;249(1):195–202.
7. van Rhijn BWG, van der Poel HG, van der Kwast TH. Urine markers for bladder cancer surveillance: a systematic review. Eur Urol. 2005;47(6):736–48.

Chapter 6
Haematospermia

Nicholas Raison and Ben Challacombe

Haematospermia, or haemospermia, is defined as the presence of fresh or altered blood in the ejaculate. It has been recognised for centuries by others such as Hippocrates, Galen and Fournier although the historical associations with "unbridled licence" and "excessive overindulgence" no longer form the focus of investigation.

For patients haematospermia can be a disconcerting symptom that often occurs acutely without warning and triggers considerable anxiety. A decade ago, up to 70 % would be diagnosed as idiopathic. Nowadays with the development of accurate, non-invasive imaging, a cause is found in 85 % of cases [1] although thankfully most cases are self limiting and not related to underlying malignancy.

An extensive number of aetiologies have been described but the most common are iatrogenic trauma such as prostate biopsy and infection or inflammation particularly in patients

N. Raison (✉)
Department of Urology, Guy's and St. Thomas NHS
Foundation Trust, London, UK
e-mail: nicholasraison@googlemail.com

B. Challacombe
Department of Urology, Guy's and St. Thomas NHS
Foundation Trust, Great Maze Pond, London SE1 9RT, UK
e-mail: benchallacombe@doctors.org.uk

B. Challacombe, S. Bott (eds.), *Diagnostic Techniques in Urology*,   49
DOI 10.1007/978-1-4471-2766-6_6,
© Springer-Verlag London 2014

under 40. Malignant tumours, principally prostate, testicular and seminal vesicle cancers, constitute rare but important differentials that must also be excluded [2]. Likewise bladder tumours situated at the bladder neck can bleed when the bladder neck contracts at the point of ejaculation leading to haematospermia.

Haematospermia is most prevalent in younger men under the age of 40 (mean age of presentation is 37 years) for whom it is generally a benign and self-limiting that necessitates minimal investigations [3]. For older patients or those with risk factors or associated symptoms, there is an association with serious underlying pathological that warrants more extensive investigation.

History

Firstly it is important to differentiate true from pseudo-haematospermia.

Other sources of blood such as haematuria or post coital bleeding caused by gynaecological disease, anorectal pathology or vaginal microtears can easily be mistaken for haematospermia. When in doubt the "condom test" can be used whereby ejaculate from within a condom is collected, and haemorrhage on the surface of the condom can be easily identified.

To help narrow the differential diagnosis a focussed history is vital. The amount, colour, frequency and duration of haematospermia should be established. Persistent haematospermia is defined as either continuous or recurrent. The colour may help differentiate urethral bleeding (bright red/pink) from causes within the prostate or seminal vesicles, that give darker, altered blood. Discolouration of the semen may be due to other reasons such as pyospermia (stained yellow) or melanspermia, a rare presentation of metastatic melanoma. Associated symptoms such as pain and storage bladder symptoms are important to establish as they can indicate an inflammatory process.

A full medical history must also be taken asking specifically about previous pelvic, genital or perineal trauma (including surgery such as urethral instrumentation or haemorrhoid operations), the presence of systemic symptoms (fever, weight loss) and any history of hypertension or bleeding diathesis. A sexual history, travel history (with emphasis on exposure to TB or schistosomiasis) and drug history particularly anticoagulant or anti platelet use should also be recorded. A history of smoking or of exposure to occupational carcinogens should also be undertaken.

Like the history, the physical examination needs to be systematic and focussed to exclude systemic and local pathology. Measure the blood pressure (malignant hypertension is a rare cause) and palpate the abdomen for pelvic masses and hepatosplenomegaly. Make a detailed assessment of the external genitalia, perineum and groin looking signs of inflammation, infection, masses or skin lesions that may cause bleeding. Identify the testis and spermatic cord, palpating the vasa for an induration or nodularity. Digital rectal examination (DRE) should assess the rectum, prostate and seminal vesicles for masses, cysts and prostatitis. After the DRE is important to recheck the meatus for blood.

Investigations

Basic laboratory tests include full blood count and coagulation screen to exclude coagulation disorders and establish the extent of bleeding. Serum prostatic specific antigen (PSA) should be considered in men over 40 years. Clean catch urine and ejaculate analysis and bacterial culture should be routinely performed with additional staining for TB or parasites if indicated by the history. If prostatitis is suspected, expressed prostatic secretions should also be sent for microbiological analysis. Screening for sexual transmitted infections and urethral swabs should be performed in all at risk patients.

Imaging

Transrectal Ultrasound (TRUS)

Transrectal Ultrasound (TRUS) is the primary imaging modality for investigating haematospermia [4]. It is a safe, inexpensive, widely available and provides detailed, high resolution images of the prostate gland, seminal vesicles, ejaculatory ducts and ampullary portions of the vas deferens. Additionally to aid diagnosis TRUS guided aspiration or biopsy of the seminal vesicles or prostate may be performed.

Scrotal Ultrasound

Scrotal ultrasound should be considered in younger patients presenting with unexplained recurrent or persistent haematospermia to exclude testicular neoplasia, a rare but significant differential.

Magnetic Resonance Imaging

Magnetic Resonance Imaging (MRI) with an endorectal coil is the gold standard for imaging the ejaculatory ducts, ampullary vas, vermontanum and internal architecture of the prostate [2]. It has excellent soft tissue contrast in particular for detecting haemorrhage, and has been shown to be more sensitive than TRUS. MRI therefore provides an important second line modality if TRUS is not satisfactory.

Vasovesical Vesiculography

Vasovesical vesiculography is rarely used for evaluating haematospermia but can aid diagnosis of aplastic or obstructed ejaculatory ducts. It is performed by exposuring the vas deferens through a scrotal incision and cannulated with a 23G needle and contrast is then injected up the vas with plain frontal pelvic radiographs are taken. This is rarely required and only performed in specialist andrological centres.

Computed Tomography

Computed Tomography can identify calcifications, gross soft tissue masses, and cystic lesions of the prostate or ejaculatory ducts. But the poor differentiation of small calibre structures or the internal architecture of the prostate in comparison to TRUS and Endorectal MRU limits its use.

Cystoscopy

Cystoscopy provides direct visualisation of the prostatic urethra, bladder neck and bladder to identify urethritis, urethral polyps, calculi, vascular anomalies or foreign bodies, which may otherwise be missed. Flexible cystoscopy is generally preferable to rigid cystoscopy since it can be performed under local anaesthesia and retroflexion allows visualisation of the bladder neck to identify tumours and potential varicosities. A drawback of cystoscopy is that intermittent bleeding is easily missed and is many distended veins are only visible during erection. This can be overcome by inducing an erection during flexible cystoscopy and using prostatic massage to stimulate bleeding.

Investigation Summary

Baseline:

- Blood Pressure measurement
- Urine Dipstick/Mid-stream Urine for culture
- PSA
- Semen Culture
- Flexible cystoscopy
- If associated micro/macro haematuria

Persistent Symptoms:

- Trans Rectal Ultrasound
- Pelvic/Prostate MRI
- Scrotal Ultrasound

Management

There is no specific treatment for haematospermia which, when required, depends on the underlying condition. Management of haematospermia centres on the age, duration of haematospermia and the presence of associated symptoms of risk factors. In young patient under 40 years, the aetiology is likely to be infectious and sexual transmitted infections should be excluded. However if haematuria resolves, further investigation and imaging is not required. In the majority of cases, bleeding is minimal and self-limiting and can be managed expectantly. The most important aspect of management is then to reassure the patient and address common concerns such as fertility or sexual function.

In older patients or if there are concerning features in the history or examination, a more extensive investigation is required. Patients should have their PSA measured (if over 40 years) and undergo TRUS. Flexible cystoscopy should also be considered especially if there is any history of haematuria, lower urinary tract symptoms or risk factors for transitional cell carcinoma of the baldder. Negative TRUS necessitates endorectal MRI.

References

1. Papp GK, Kopa Z, Szabó F, Erdei E. Aetiology of haemospermia. Andrologia.2003;35(5):317–20.doi:10.1046/j.1439-0272.2003.00575.x.
2. Ahmad I, Krishna NS. Hemospermia. J Urol. 2007;177(5):1613–8. doi:10.1016/j.juro.2007.01.004.
3. Mulhall JP, Albertsen PC. Hemospermia: diagnosis and management. Urology. 1995;46(4):463–7.
4. Zhao H, Luo J, Wang D, et al. The value of transrectal ultrasound in the diagnosis of hematospermia in a large cohort of patients. J Androl. 2012;33(5):897–903. doi:10.2164/jandrol.111.013318.

Chapter 7
Diagnostic Techniques in Male LUTS/BPE

Faith McMeekin and Mark J. Speakman

Lower urinary tract symptoms (LUTS) were traditionally attributed to the enlarging prostate alone. We know however that there is an important interplay between LUTS, benign prostate enlargement (BPE) and bladder outlet obstruction (BOO) [1]. In addition there are important effects from the urethra, the bladder and both the peripheral and central nervous systems, as well as non-urological causes of LUTS. These non-urological causes include renal, endocrine, neurological and cardiac causes that can influence these symptoms. Despite the numerous underlying causes of LUTS, the focus of this chapter will be to cover the diagnostic tests that have a role in quantifying the symptoms and diagnosing BOO as a result of BPE.

It is important when taking a history from a male patient with LUTS to establish whether they are predominantly storage, voiding or post micturition symptoms (see Table 7.1) and most importantly how "bothersome" these symptoms are to the patient's quality of life (QoL).

F. McMeekin, MBBS, BSc, MRCS • M.J. Speakman, MS, FRCS (✉)
Department of Urology, Musgrove Park Hospital,
Taunton and Somerset NHS Foundation Trust, Taunton, UK
e-mail: mark.speakman@tst.nhs.uk

B. Challacombe, S. Bott (eds.), *Diagnostic Techniques in Urology*,   55
DOI 10.1007/978-1-4471-2766-6_7,
© Springer-Verlag London 2014

TABLE 7.1 Symptom categories

Storage symptoms	Voiding symptoms	Post-micturition symptoms
Altered bladder sensation	Hesitancy	Sensation of incomplete emptying
Increased daytime frequency	Intermittency	Post micturition dribble
Nocturia	Slow stream	
Urgency	Splitting/spraying	
Urinary incontinence	Straining	
	Terminal dribble	

For patients presenting with suspected urological LUTS a simple flowchart (Fig. 7.1) is presented for assessment and subsequent investigation and diagnosis. In this chapter we will cover each section in more detail, highlighting when certain investigations should be considered.

History

This is the most important aspect of patient assessment and should include as a minimum:

- *Symptoms* – duration, extent and impact on QoL
- *Lifestyle* – fluid intake and type
- *Medications/drugs* – any previously tried/current medications for any condition
- *Past medical history* – previous pelvic surgery, trauma, neurological disorders

As an adjunct to the history completion of an International Prostate Scoring System (IPSS) will act not only to quantify symptoms, but also act as a comparison following treatment [2]. The validated questionnaire consists of seven questions, scored 0–5, based on the extent of symptoms and a single quality-of-life question (QOL) to assess how troublesome the symptoms

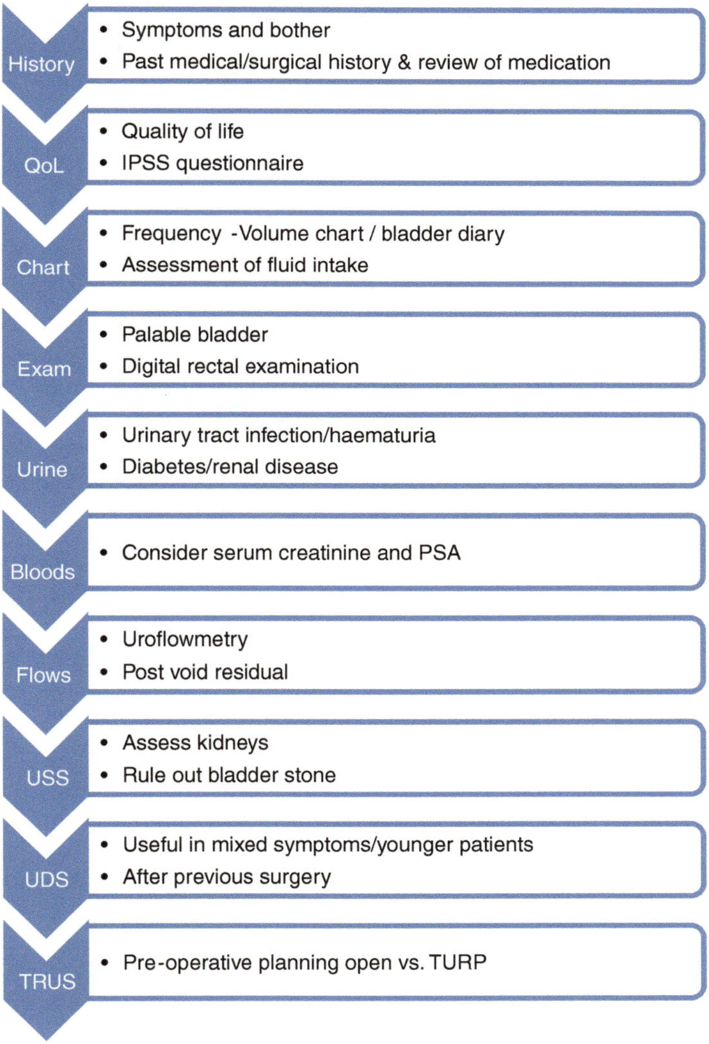

History
- Symptoms and bother
- Past medical/surgical history & review of medication

QoL
- Quality of life
- IPSS questionnaire

Chart
- Frequency -Volume chart / bladder diary
- Assessment of fluid intake

Exam
- Palable bladder
- Digital rectal examination

Urine
- Urinary tract infection/haematuria
- Diabetes/renal disease

Bloods
- Consider serum creatinine and PSA

Flows
- Uroflowmetry
- Post void residual

USS
- Assess kidneys
- Rule out bladder stone

UDS
- Useful in mixed symptoms/younger patients
- After previous surgery

TRUS
- Pre-operative planning open vs. TURP

FIGURE 7.1 Flowchart for assessment and investigation for a patient presenting with LUTS

are to the patient. On the basis of the answers to the individual questions a total score is obtained which can be used to divide patients into three categories. Mild LUTS is defined as a score of 0–7, moderate 8–19 and severe LUTS 20–35. The QoL question is scored 0–6, where 6 is most bothersome.

Frequency-Volume Chart

In addition to the IPSS, a more useful marker of bladder activity is a frequency- volume chart or bladder diary. The patient should complete a minimum 3-day diary highlighting timing and volume of voids, including any episodes of incontinence throughout the 72-h period. It is the most accurate tool in diagnosing nocturnal polyuria. This is calculated by adding the volume of all voids overnight including the first void of the morning and dividing it by the total voided volume in that 24 h. If this is greater than a third then nocturnal polyuria is diagnosed and a variety of alternate treatments such as an afternoon diuretic or desmopression need to be considered to shift the diuresis to avoid disturbed sleep.

Examination

Abdominal examination should include examination for an enlarged bladder (chronic retention) by percussing the bladder. The external genitalia and the foreskin should also be carefully examined. Digital rectal examination is done to detect abnormalities, which may indicate an underlying prostate cancer. In addition it provides an approximation of prostate size.

Urinanalysis

This is a useful simple cheap test that all patients presenting with urological symptoms should have performed. The urine dipstick analyses the following components

pH – The average urinary pH is between 5.5 and 6.5. An alkaline pH in the presence of UTI suggests the possibility of renal tract stones. Certain bacterial organisms produce an enzyme that produces ammonia which raises the pH of the urine and this can precipitate magnesium ammonium phosphate to form staghorn stones.

Blood – normal urine contains <3 RBCs per high-powered field. A positive dipstick for blood indicates the presence of haemoglobin in the urine which has a sensitivity of >90 %

Protein – this is usually secondary to renal disease. Normal adults have a urinary protein concentration <20 mg/dL, anything greater than this shows positive on dipstick testing, >20mg/dL results in green discoloration of tetrabromophenolblue dye.

Leucocytes – white blood cells in the urine produce the enzyme leucocyte esterase and this causes a colour change in a chromogen salt on the dipstick.

Nitrites – most gram-negative bacteria, which are the commonest urinary pathogens, convert nitrates, normally present in the urine, to nitrites which are not normally present. These nitrites react with the reagent on the dipstick to form a red/pink azo dye reaction called the '***Greiss reaction***'.

Urine microscopy – all urine samples historically used to be viewed under the microscope to identify organisms, but now more routinely samples undergo flow cytometry to establish if cell counts are indicative of infection prior to microscopy and culture. If flow cytometry is positive then samples are cultured on blood agar plates and subsequent sensitivities are established.

Blood Tests

In initial investigation these should be reserved for selected patients. Perform a baseline serum creatinine only if there is a suspicion of renal impairment [3] particularly if there is a possibility of high pressure chronic retention causing renal dysfunction i.e. large post void bladder residual volumes associated with nocturnal incontinence.

In addition if size matters, as it appears to do, a prostate specific antigen (PSA) test as a proxy for volume and a risk factor for progression may be useful in the management of benign prostatic disease. Although a provocative suggestion, a single PSA may be of greater value in managing benign prostate disease than in managing and diagnosing malignant prostate disease, where sequential testing is more important.

Uroflowmetry

Measurement of a patient's flow rate provides a visual image of the '*strength*' of their urinary stream. It is measured in ml/s using electronic flow meters, which provide a printout recording the voided volume, maximum flow rate, and time taken to complete the void, together with a printed visual record of the flow pattern. Maximum flow rate (Qmax) is influenced by the volume of urine voided, contractility of the patients' bladder and the resistance of their urethra. It is for this reason that the flow test can reveal evidence of bladder outflow obstruction and with experience one can estimate the most likely underlying cause; BPE, urethral stricture or detrusor failure and this is most easily recognised by the 'pattern' of the flow curve. Although urine flow rate can be useful in diagnosis it does not predict outcome of treatment; a large Veterans Administration trial compared conservative treatment and TURP and found that flow rate could not predict the likelihood of a good symptomatic outcome after TURP [4] (Fig. 7.2).

Ultrasound

This is a non-invasive method of imaging the urinary tract; it is particularly good for providing anatomical information of the kidneys and bladder. For men with urinary retention, particularly high volume retention it is useful to evaluate

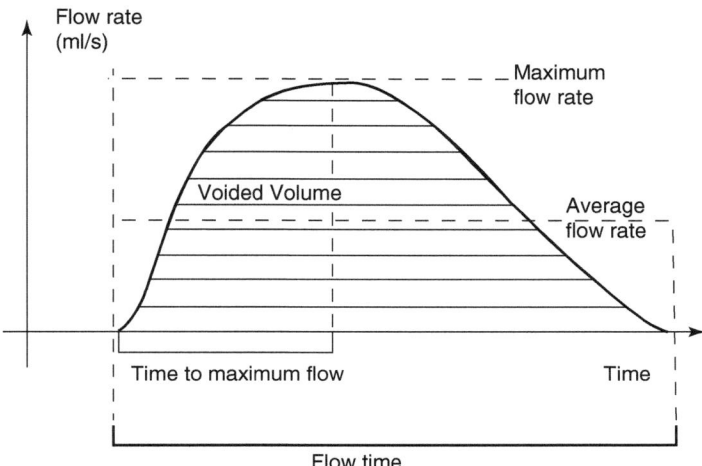

FIGURE 7.2 Terminology relating to the description of urinary flow (ICS report [5])

if there is evidence of hydronephrosis secondary to high pressure chronic retention as this requires urgent decompression with catheterisation. If chronic retention presents with an elevated creatinine an urgent USS is required.

The USS will also identify any underlying bladder cause for LUTS, such as a bladder stone or large bladder tumour. Although it is not used traditionally to establish prostate size trans-abdominally there can be suggestions of an enlarged prostate with indentation of the bladder wall, further heightening suspicion that this may be the underlying cause of the patient's LUTS.

To accurately assess prostate volume a transrectal US scan (TRUSS) is required. This utilises a probe, inserted via the rectum and taking height, width and length measurements in two planes producing an accurate calculation of prostate volume. This is useful when planning surgery, as volumes in excess of 100 cc can be considered for open Millen's prostatectomy or Holmium enucleation.

Urodynamics

This should not be considered a routine investigation for patients presenting with LUTS. It should however be considered for patients before surgery who present at a younger or considerably older age, those with underlying neurological diseases and in those who have had previous surgery that has failed or in those who have had a recurrence of symptoms. It might also be considered in those where have failed conservative management and in whom it is not clear from their symptom complex or flow test whether they have obstruction or not.

UDS measure flow and pressure during filling and voiding. This is achieved by placing a line into a patient's bladder, which is connected to a transducer, together with another line placed rectally (mimicking abdominal pressure). Subtracting the two will give a true detrusor pressure, which can be measured throughout filling and voiding to assess if there is evidence of bladder outflow obstruction and or detrusor over/underactivity.

Typically for patients with BOO secondary to BPE there is high detrusor pressure on voiding; this in combination with a poor flow gives an elevated bladder outflow obstruction index (BOOI). Where **BOOI = pdetQmax − 2Qmax. pdetQmax is** detrusor pressure at maximum flow rate.

BOOI >40 = Obstructed
BOOI 20–40 = Equivocal
BOOI <20 = Unobstructed

There are a wide variety of diagnostic investigations that are available for male LUTS. It is important to recognise, throughout every patient assessment, the impact LUTS have on a patient's life. Arguably the most valuable aspects are a good history and the QoL question on the IPSS in planning subsequent investigations. It may be that the patient requires reassurance, lifestyle advice/modification as their symptoms cause minimal "bother". However if a patient has troublesome symptoms then baseline assessment should include

DRE, urinanalysis, frequency/volume chart, and consideration of PSA/creatinine and a urinary flow test with post void residual which will guide further evaluation and treatment.

References

1. Abrams P, Cardozo L, Fall M, Griffiths D, Rosier P, Ulmsten U, et al. The standardisation of terminology in lower urinary tract function: report from the standardisation sub-committee of the International Continence Society. Urology. 2003;61(1):37–49.
2. Barry MJ, Fowler FJ, O'Leary MP, Bruskewitz RC, Holtgrewe HL, Mebust WK, et al. The American Urological Association symptom index for benign prostatic hyperplasia. The Measurement Committee of the American Urological Association. J Urol. 1992;148(5): 1549–57. discussion 64.
3. Jones C, Hill J, Chapple C, Group GD. Management of lower urinary tract symptoms in men: summary of NICE guidance. BMJ. 2010;340:c2354.
4. Bruskewitz RC, Reda DJ, Wasson JH, Barrett L, Phelan M. Testing to predict outcome after transurethral resection of the prostate. J Urol. 1997;157(4):1304–8.
5. Griffiths D, Höfner K, van Mastrigt R, Rollema HJ, Spångberg A, Gleason D. Standardization of terminology of lower urinary tract function: pressure-flow studies of voiding, urethral resistance, and urethral obstruction. International Continence Society Subcommittee on Standardization of Terminology of Pressure-Flow Studies. Neurourol Urodyn. 1997;16(1):1–18.

Chapter 8
Storage Lower Urinary Tract Symptoms: Evaluation and Investigations

Jai Seth, Arun Sahai, and Prokar Dasgupta

Introduction

The role of the lower urinary tract is to store urine, at low pressures, and to allow voiding at appropriate times. To regulate this, a complex neural network exists which acts in a switch like manner to balance the bladder reservoir and the sphincteric tap. A variety of lower urinary tract pathology can lead to the experience of lower urinary tract symptoms (LUTS), due to benign or neoplastic conditions affecting the bladder, prostate or urethra. These symptoms can be categorized into three main divisions, such as storage, voiding and post-micturition symptoms. This chapter focuses on storage LUTS, which accompany the overactive bladder (OAB).

Lower urinary tract symptoms in general are highly prevalent, with symptoms of overactive bladder thought to affect up to 17 % of men and women [1]. OAB syndrome as defined by the International Continence Society (ICS) is a syndrome of storage symptoms: essentially urinary urgency, with or without urgency incontinence, usually associated

J. Seth, BSc, MSc, MRCS
A. Sahai, PhD, FRCS (Urol), BSc (Hons) (✉)
P. Dasgupta, MSc, MD, FRCS (Urol), FEBU
Department of Urology, Guy's Hospital NHS Foundation Trust and King's College London School of Medicine, London, UK
e-mail: sonnyroth@yahoo.com

B. Challacombe, S. Bott (eds.), *Diagnostic Techniques in Urology*, 65
DOI 10.1007/978-1-4471-2766-6_8,
© Springer-Verlag London 2014

with daytime frequency and nocturia in the absence of any other pathology. Associated with this, the patient may have a reduced interval between voids and a reduced volume voided per micturition [2]. Urgency refers to an abnormal or sudden inappropriate compelling desire to void, which is very difficult to defer for fear of urinary leakage. This is to be differentiated from the normal sensations of bladder filling, which progressively are the first sensation of filling (FSF), first desire to void (FDV) and strong desire to void (SDV), and these can be measured and demonstrated during a urodynamic study [2]. Whilst presenting a large health and economic burden, OAB syndrome remains underdiagnosed and undertreated. The prevalence increases with age, especially in those over 60 years of age, and although up to 60 % of older patients seek treatment, only 27 % receive it [1].

Irwin et al. estimated from the EPIC study the economic impact of OAB. Data from the UK estimates that each OAB patient per annum has 'excess direct costs' of €515 (including medical consultation €225, clinical depression €204, incontinence pad use €48 and prescription costs €33), direct costs of €13 (such as urinary tract infections [UTIs]) and nursing home costs of €381 [3]. Overall in the UK there are direct costs of €1.007 billion of direct costs associated with OAB, €579 million of nursing home costs and €233 million of lost productivity costs [3].

Although the underlying pathophysiology of OAB is largely unknown and is thought to be multifactorial, it has been shown that certain sensory neurotransmitter substances are upregulated, hence leading to the burden of urgency [4]. Physiologically, there appears to be a combination of a lower sensory threshold of bladder afferent nerve firing, an increased sensitivity to contractile transmitters, an immaturity of the central inhibitory pathways controlling micturition and potentially an intrinsic detrusor muscle problem. OAB can be classified as either idiopathic OAB, or maybe associated with urinary tract infection, bladder outflow obstruction (BOO) due to benign or malignant prostatic enlargement, neurological pathology such as spinal cord injury and multiple sclerosis which leads to neurogenic detrusor overactivity (DO), pelvic organ prolapsed and inflammatory and neoplastic bladder conditions [5, 6].

Evaluation

There may be no obvious clinical signs on examination, hence the cornerstone of evaluation involves information taken from history, which is supplemented by a bladder diary. Patients may complain of urgency, frequency (worse than their normal habit ie an increase in daytime frequency), nocturia (waking up to void once or more times at night after falling asleep) [1]. This may or may not be associated with urge incontinence.

An examination should be performed of the abdomen and pelvis to exclude any pelvic masses and any benign or malignant prostatic enlargement. A neurological examination should be carried out to exclude any deficit, which may be due to an underlying neurological pathology. A urine dipstick analysis should be taken to exclude the presence of a urinary tract infection (UTI), and a sample sent for microscopy, culture and sensitivity [7]. Any detected haematuria or recurrent UTI should be investigated appropriately.

Symptoms should be further assessed with the use of a 72 h voiding diary [8]. This simple tool, its use supported by NICE and the EAU, allows the patient to record the volume and timings of fluid intake. A high fluid intake at night for example may be of particular importance in patients who have troublesome nocturia. This can also assess the nature of fluids such as caffeine and alcohol, which can cause a diuresis and worsen bladder symptoms. The diary will demonstrate the frequency of day and night-time voids, and episodes of leakage can also be documented, which can vary from a few drops to light or heavy leaks. If >33 % of the 24 h urine volume is at night-time, between 24.00 and 08.00, then this is referred to as nocturnal polyuria, which can worsen bladder symptoms at night, and have different implications for treatment [9]. The typical patient with OAB will have frequent voids during the day and night. The voided volumes may vary as the underlying detrusor may contract erroneously at variable degrees of distension, well before maximum capacity, without warning to the patient.

Questionnaire based tools can be used to objectively assess and quantify severity of symptoms, and the knock on effects on quality of life [10], and are increasingly used by clinicians in both general practice and secondary care. Validated questionnaires include the International Consultation on Incontinence Modular Questionnaires (ICIQS), which provide different types of questionnaire, which address the range of LUTS [10, 11]. Other popular validated tools include the King's Health Questionnaire (KHQ), Urinary Symptom Profile (USP), International Prostate Symptom score (IPSS), Urogenital Distress Inventory-6 (UDI-6) and the Incontinence Impact Questionnaire (IIQ). Some of these go on to assess affects on social interaction, sleep, concern, bother and coping skills.

Investigations

Patients should receive a uroflowometry assessment, with a minimum voided volume of 150 ml, to assess the maximum speed and pattern of urination. It is preferable to obtain at least 2–3 recordings on different occasions rather based decisions on a one off result. Ultrasound measurements of estimated post-void residuals should be performed on multiple occasions, to ascertain whether the patient has difficulty emptying the bladder. This is important as incomplete bladder emptying and OAB can co-exist, and furthermore OAB can be secondary to BOO. Detrusor underactivity can also contribute to poor voiding and lead to high post-void residual volumes [7]. A more formal ultrasound can also be performed to assess for other causes of urgency such as pelvic masses or urolithiasis [12].

Male patients may incorrectly associate LUTS with prostate cancer. Prostate-specific antigen (PSA) testing can be offered to patients at their request and after appropriate counselling regarding its benefits and limitations. Prostate cancer screening is currently under debate and large studies from the USA and Europe have provided conflicting information [13, 14]. Patients with an abnormal PSA result or abnormal feeling prostate on rectal examination should be referred for further assessment in accordance with EAU guidance [15]. Once patients have attempted initial conservative methods of treatment, including lifestyle and dietary modifications, and have proved to be resistant to first line antimuscarinic medications, then more sophisticated assessments of the bladder can be performed. These will initially involve urodynamics, but in certain cases videourodynamics and neurophysiological outpatient studies maybe warranted. Although these investigations are more invasive they can provide more accurate information of the bladder and urethral sphincter function during filling and voiding. Whilst OAB is a symptomatic diagnosis, these symptoms are associated with urodynamically demonstrable unstable detrusor contractions (detrsuor overactivity), which are evident in 76.1 and 58.7 % of male and female patients with OAB respectively. This correlation is even stronger in those who have urgency incontinence with incidence of 93 and 69.8 % of men and women respectively [16]. A urodynamic study in an incontinent patient can also identify, if there is a stress incontinence component to their symptoms which would influence the path of treatment considered. The study will also provide information regarding the maximum bladder capacity, and the volume at the first sensation of filling (FSF), the first desire to void (FDV) and the sudden desire to void (SDV). Furthermore when analyzing the voiding phase clear evidence of BOO can be demonstrated based on the ICS nomogram [17].

A videourodynamic study can also provide additional anatomical information and give a more dynamic assessment of the bladder. This is particularly relevant when assessing neurological bladders or those who have had prior surgery to treat their symptoms/incontinence. In addition these studies can identify vesico-ureteric reflux and look at the bladder neck for descent. A summary of this evaluation and investigation pathway can be seen in Fig. 8.1.

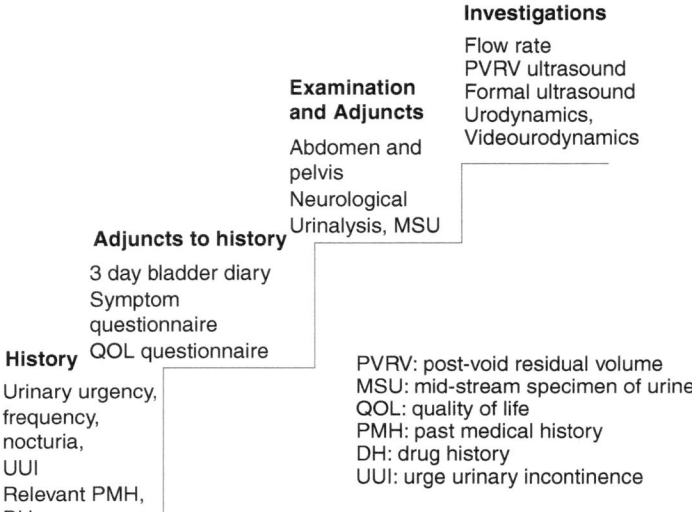

FIGURE 8.1 A summary of the evaluation of a patient with storage LUTS

Summary

The role of lower urinary tract is to store urine at low pressures, and it remains within this storage phase for 99.8 % of the time, whilst allowing appropriate voiding. The aims of evaluation and investigation of LUTS is to establish the severity of symptoms, with an indication of the knock-on effects these may have on the patient's QOL. The cause of the symptoms should be sought and any underlying sinister causes should also be detected and urgently referred on for suitable treatment. The goal of treatment would then be to improve symptoms, improve the bladder's storage capacity, and to eliminate the urgency and frequency of voiding and incontinence, whilst keeping drug side effects to a minimum. Due to the irritative nature of this condition, many therapeutic options that are implemented do have a significant improvement for quality of life and patient outcome.

Acknowledgement   Arun Sahai and Prokar Dasgupta acknowledge financial support from the Department of Health via the National Institute for Health Research (NIHR) comprehensive Biomedical Research Centre award to Guy's & St Thomas' NHS Foundation Trust in partnership with King's College London and King's College Hospital NHS Foundation Trust. They also acknowledges the support of the MRC Centre for Transplantation.

References

1. Marinkovic SP et al. The management of overactive bladder syndrome. BMJ. 2012;344:e2365.
2. Abrams P et al. The standardisation of terminology of lower urinary tract function: report from the Standardisation Sub-committee of the International Continence Society. Neurourol Urodyn. 2002;21(2):167–78.
3. Irwin DE et al. The economic impact of overactive bladder syndrome in six Western countries. BJU Int. 2009;103(2):202–9.
4. Michel MC, Chapple CR. Basic mechanisms of urgency: roles and benefits of pharmacotherapy. World J Urol. 2009;27(6): 705–9.
5. Morant SV et al. Diagnosis and treatment of lower urinary tract symptoms suggestive of overactive bladder and bladder outlet obstruction among men in general practice in the UK. Int J Clin Pract. 2008;62(5):688–94.
6. Panicker JN, de Seze M, Fowler CJ. Rehabilitation in practice: neurogenic lower urinary tract dysfunction and its management. Clin Rehabil. 2010;24(7):579–89.
7. Foon R, Drake MJ. The overactive bladder. Ther Adv Urol. 2010;2(4):147–55.
8. Abrams P, Klevmark B. Frequency volume charts: an indispensable part of lower urinary tract assessment. Scand J Urol Nephrol Suppl. 1996;179:47–53.
9. Rembratt A, Norgaard JP, Andersson KE. What is nocturnal polyuria? BJU Int. 2002;90 Suppl 3:18–20.
10. Irwin DE et al. Population-based survey of urinary incontinence, overactive bladder, and other lower urinary tract symptoms in five countries: results of the EPIC study. Eur Urol. 2006;50(6): 1306–14; discussion 1314–5.

11. Abrams P et al. The International Consultation on Incontinence Modular Questionnaire: www.iciq.net. J Urol. 2006;175(3 Pt 1):1063–6; discussion 1066.

12. Thuroff JW et al. EAU guidelines on urinary incontinence. Eur Urol. 2011;59(3):387–400.

13. Andriole GL et al. Mortality results from a randomized prostate-cancer screening trial. N Engl J Med. 2009;360(13):1310–9.

14. Schroder FH et al. Screening and prostate-cancer mortality in a randomized European study. N Engl J Med. 2009;360(13):1320–8.

15. Heidenreich A, Bastian PJ, Bellmunt J, Joniau S, Bolla M, Mason MD, Matveev V, Mottet N, Wiegel T, van der Kwast TH, Zattoni F. Guidelines on prostate cancer. Eur Assoc Urol. 2012.

16. Al-Ghazo MA et al. Urodynamic detrusor overactivity in patients with overactive bladder symptoms. Int Neurourol J. 2011;15(1):48–54.

17. Abrams P. Bladder outlet obstruction index, bladder contractility index and bladder voiding efficiency: three simple indices to define bladder voiding function. BJU Int. 1999;84(1):14–5.

Chapter 9
Urinary Incontinence

Melissa C. Davies and Tamsin Drake

Definitions [1]

Urinary Incontinence	The complaint of any involuntary leakage of urine
Stress Urinary Incontinence (SUI)	The complaint of involuntary leakage of urine on effort or exertion, or on sneezing or coughing.
Urodynamic Stress Incontinence (USI)	The involuntary leakage of urine when there is a rise in abdominal pressure (induced by coughing or straining) during filling cystometry, in the absence of a detrusor contraction.

M.C. Davies (✉) • T. Drake, BM, MRCS
Department of Urology, Salisbury District Hospital, Salisbury, UK
e-mail: melissa.davies@salisbury.nhs.uk; tamsindrake@hotmail.com

B. Challacombe, S. Bott (eds.), *Diagnostic Techniques in Urology*,   73
DOI 10.1007/978-1-4471-2766-6_9,
© Springer-Verlag London 2014

Urge Urinary Incontinence (UUI)	The complaint of any involuntary leakage of urine accompanied by or immediate preceded by the urgency to void.
Overactive Bladder	The complaint of urgency, with or without urge incontinence, usually with frequency and nocturia.
Mixed Urinary Incontinence (MUI)	A combination of SUI and UUI.
Overflow Urinary Incontinence	The complaint of involuntary leakage of urine when the bladder is abnormally distended with large post-void residuals.
Nocturnal enuresis	The complaint of loss of urine during sleep.
Post-micturition dribble	The complaint of a dribbling loss of urine after voiding, predominantly affecting males due to pooling of urine in the bulbar urethra.

Introduction

Urinary incontinence (UI) is the complaint of any involuntary leakage of urine [1]. This leakage of urine may be urethral or extra-urethral (secondary to anatomical abnormalities such as fistulae and ectopic ureters). It is an extremely common condition worldwide, and it is likely that all practicing doctors and nurses will come into contact with patients with this problem at some point during their careers.

UI has the potential to cause a great deal of psychosocial harm, as well as posing a significant financial burden on both affected individuals and society. Overall, the annual incidence of UI in women ranges from 2 to 11 %, with the highest incidence occurring during pregnancy [2]. Corresponding literature for the overall incidence of UI among men is scarce, however the figure is widely accepted as being lower than in women.

Stress urinary incontinence (SUI) is the most common type of UI in women, affecting 1 in 4 of the female population, and increasing with increasing age. It results from hypermobility of the bladder neck/pelvic floor, and/or intrinsic urethral sphincter deficiency. Stress incontinence can be confirmed on urodynamic testing, after which it is referred to as "urodynamic stress incontinence". Video-urodynamics help to further classify the condition into types 0–III according to the appearances of the bladder neck and/or proximal urethra during stress-induced urinary leakages.

Urge urinary incontinence (UUI) is less prevalent than SUI but appears to affect males and females equally. When demonstrated on urodynamic testing, the term "detrusor overactivity incontinence" is used.

Many patients will have both patterns of incontinence, and the aim is to establish the predominant pattern in order to obtain the best treatment outcomes.

History

A full and detailed history is probably the most useful tool in assessing patients with urinary incontinence. This can be supplemented with the use of validated questionnaires, such as ICIQ-SF (International Consultation on Incontinence Questionnaire Short Form) [3]. These questionnaires can then be repeated following any intervention for urinary incontinence, as a more objective measure of how successful treatment has been. Voiding diaries (also known as micturition time charts, frequency/volume charts and bladder diaries) allow quantification of variables such voided volume, likely bladder capacity and nocturnal urine output.

Taking a careful clinical history should allow the patient's urinary incontinence to be categorised into stress, urgency or mixed. It will also help identify patients who need prompt referral to a specialist. In females, it is important to include a detailed obstetric history including; number of births, instrumental deliveries or breech deliveries, as well as a gynaecological history. This may aid understanding of the underlying aetiology and identify factors, which may impact on treatment decisions. Other important co-morbidities which may impact on, or cause symptoms of urinary incontinence include; back problems/previous spinal surgery, neurological conditions, chronic constipation, previous pelvic surgery (including prostatectomy) and prior radiotherapy. It is also important to ascertain details of current medications that the patient is taking as some of these may lead to or exacerbate urinary incontinence (Table 9.1).

Examination

A full external examination of the patient is required. In patients of both sexes this should include:

- Abdominal examination: to identify scars from previous surgery and to elicit any bladder enlargement, or the presence of another abdominal mass
- Perineal and digital rectal examination (DRE): to assess for perianal sensation, anal tone and the presence of a faecally loaded rectum
- Simple neurological examination including a gross assessment of sensation, reflexes and muscle power in the lower limbs.
- A cough test (ideally undertaken in the standing position with a comfortably full bladder) to elicit stress incontinence.

  In men (a chaperone should be offered):

- Digital examination of the prostate

TABLE 9.1 Risk factors for urinary incontinence

Gender (F > M)
Race (Caucasian > Afro-Caribbean)
Increasing age
Genetic predisposition
Neurological disease (including spinal cord injury, stroke, multiple sclerosis, Parkinson's disease, dementia and general cognitive impairment)
Anatomical abnormalities (including urinary fistulae, ectopic ureter and urethral diverticulum)
High parity (particularly if vaginal and/or traumatic deliveries)
Previous pelvic surgery
Previous pelvic radiotherapy
Diabetes Mellitus
Chronic constipation
Obesity
Medications (including alpha blockers, calcium channel blockers, cholinergics, ACE inhibitors causing chronic cough, benzodiazepines, systemic oestrogen, antidepressants, diuretics, antihistamines, opiates)
Increased fluid intake
Poor mobility

In women (with a chaperone present):

- Inspection of the vulva and vagina looking for pink and moist mucosa suggesting healthy oestrogenisation (atrophic vaginitis will exacerbate any urinary symptoms that the patients may have, and should be treated with topical oestrogen preparations)
- An internal bimanual examination with an assessment of the pelvic floor tone

TABLE 9.2 Classifying the degree of a pelvic organ prolapse

Degree of prolapse	Appearance
First	The prolapse does not reach the introitus
Second	The prolapse protrudes through the introitus
Third	The prolapsed organ lies completely outside the introitus

TABLE 9.3 How to act upon a urine dipstick result

	Urine dip positive for leucocytes and nitrites	Urine dip positive for either leucocytes or nitrites
Symptoms of UTI	Send urine for MC&S	
	Start appropriate antibiotics (according to local microbiology guidelines) for presumed UTI, pending culture results	Consider starting appropriate antibiotics (according to local microbiology guidelines) for presumed UTI, pending culture results
No symptoms of UTI	Do not prescribe antibiotics for UTI unless the urine culture is positive	UTI unlikely; do not send urine for MC&S

- Assessment for pelvic organ prolapse
  - This is ideally performed in the left lateral position using a Sims speculum.
  - The presence and degree (see Table 9.2) of anterior, middle and posterior vaginal wall descent should be assessed (anterior vaginal prolapse may contribute significantly to urinary symptoms, and concomitant prolapse surgery may be undertaken at the same time as any surgical intervention for urinary incontinence)

Initial Investigations

Urinalysis: A urine dipstick result positive for leucocytes and/or nitrites has a low sensitivity but a high specificity for detecting urinary tract infection (UTI). Table 9.3 outlines the instances in which sending a urine sample for microscopy, culture and sensitivities (MC&S), and starting antibiotics is recommended.

Post void residual volume (PVR): this is the amount of urine that remains in the bladder after voiding. It can be determined using a bladder scanner (ultrasound) or on catheterisation. A significant PVR indicates ineffective voiding, which may be multifactorial. As such, one should be prompted to assess PVR in all patients with symptoms of voiding dysfunction and/or complicated urinary incontinence. PVR should also be monitored in patients receiving treatment that may worsen or cause voiding dysfunction e.g. Anticholinergics.

Pad test: this involves the use of a continence pad to contain urinary leakage over a period of time and therefore quantify the volume of leakage. This can be conducted over a variable length of time. Most commonly used are the 1 or 24 h pad tests.

Additional Investigations

Urodynamics: This term describes a range of tests that assess urethral and bladder function, from simple uroflowmetry to more complex ambulatory urodynamic monitoring and videourodynamics. Urodynamics should be performed where the findings may affect the choice of surgical treatment, it is not necessary to undertake these tests prior to commencing conservative management. NICE guidance does not recommend the routine use of urodynamics prior to surgical management of SUI but it is the authors recommendation that filling and voiding cystometrography be undertake prior to any surgical intervention.

In patients whom have undergone previous pelvic surgery or male patients post radical prostatectomy videourodynamics should be considered if available.

Urethrocystoscopy: This refers to the endoscopic examination of the urethra, intrinsic urethral sphincter, and bladder, this may be performed under local anaesthetic using a flexible, fibreoptic cystoscope.

Imaging: Can be used to investigate any anatomical or functional abnormalities that may be contributing to urinary incontinence. USS and MRI can both be used to provide quantitative and qualitative date on the kidneys, bladder neck and pelvic floor, but should generally be reserved for cases of "complicated" urinary incontinence.

Algorithms

The following flow charts (reproduced with permission from the 3rd International Consultation on Incontinence [4]) outline recommended pathways for the assessment and management of urinary incontinence in both primary and secondary care (Figs. 9.1, 9.2, 9.3 and 9.4).

Other Specific Types of Urinary Incontinence

Post-radical Prostatectomy Urinary Incontinence

Intrinsic sphincter weakness following radical prostatectomy (and less commonly following trans-urethral resection (TURP)) represents the commonest cause of stress urinary incontinence in men with an estimated incidence of 10–15 % [5, 6]. It is more commonly seen in men who are older at the time of their surgery, and/or have pre-existing bladder dysfunction such as detrusor overactivity.

Incontinence in the Frail and Elderly

Urinary incontinence becomes more prevalent with increasing age, particularly over the age of 70. The mnemonic "DIAPPERS" can be used as an aide memoire for the transient causes of UI in elderly patients:

Delirium
Infection

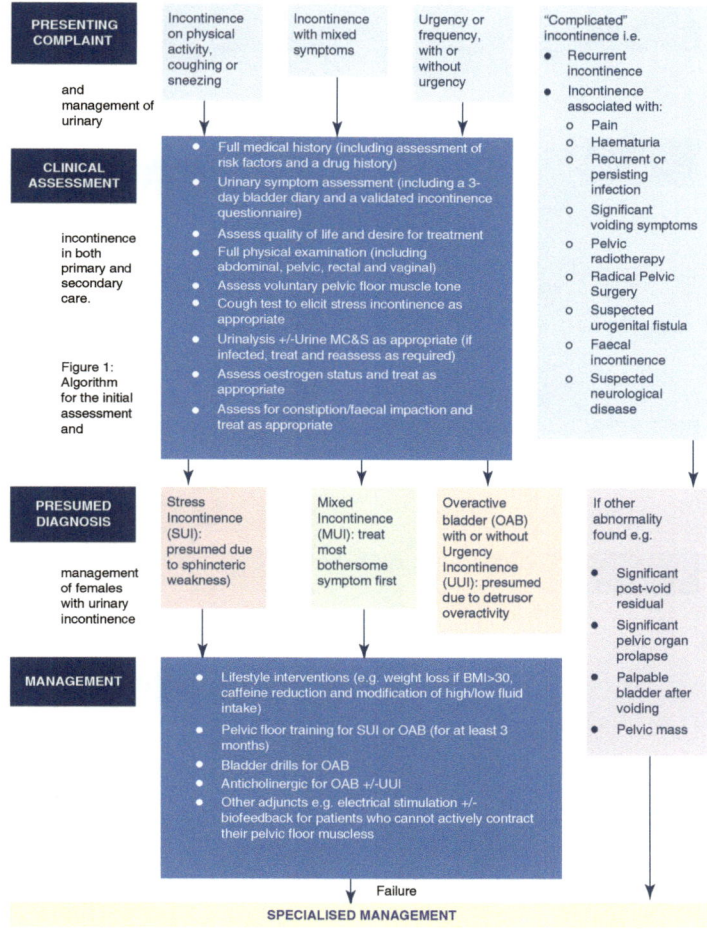

FIGURE 9.1 Algorithm for the initial assessment and management of females with urinary incontinence

Atrophic vaginitis
Pharmaceuticals (e.g. opiates, calcium channel blockers, anti-cholinergics, diuretics and alpha blockers)

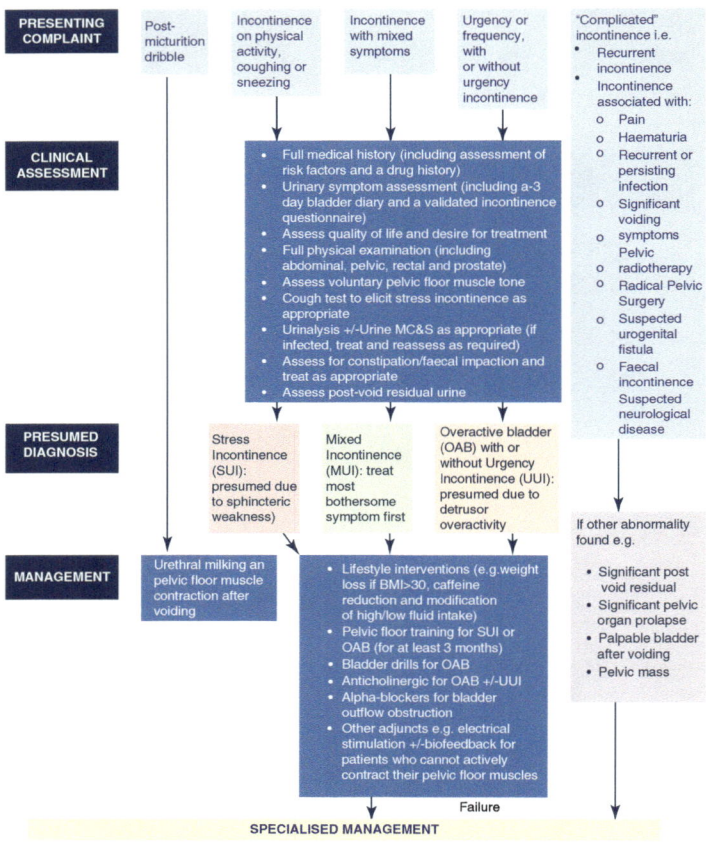

FIGURE 9.2 Algorithm for the initial assessment and management of males with urinary incontinence

Psychological problems (e.g. depression, neurosis, and anxiety)

Excess fluid input or output (e.g. due to CCF and nocturnal polyuria)

Restricted mobility

Stool impaction

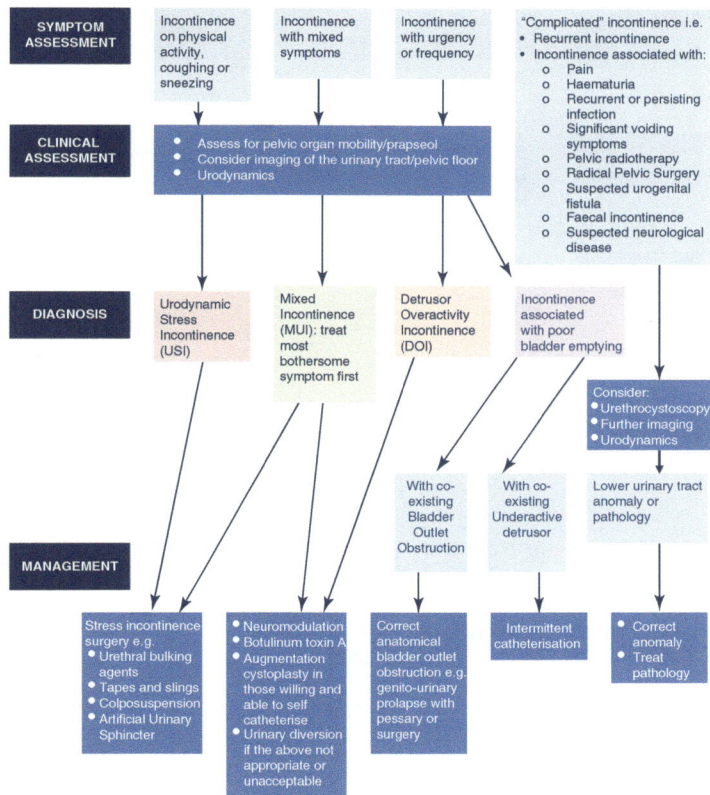

FIGURE 9.3 Algorithm for specialised management of urinary incontinence in women

Healthy and fit older persons with established UI should be offered a range of treatments, similar to those offered to their younger counterparts. However, frail older persons should be managed differently, with greater emphasis on the impact of their pre-existing co-morbidities, current medications and functional and/or cognitive impairment. Intervention in frail elderly patients should also consider how much they (and their carers) are "bothered" by their urinary incontinence, and what their overall prognosis and likely life expectancy is.

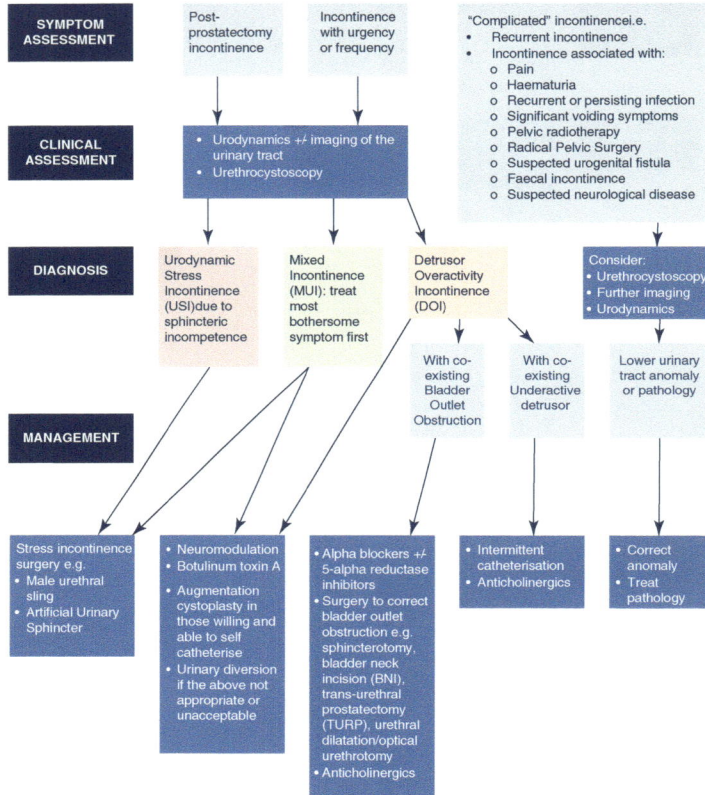

FIGURE 9.4 Algorithm for specialised management of urinary incontinence in men

References

1. Abrams P, Cardozo L, Fall M, et al. The standardization of terminology of lower urinary tract function: report from the standardization sub-committee of the International Continence Society. Neurourol Urodyn. 2002;21:167–78.
2. Wennberg AL, Molander U, Fall M, Edlund C, Peeker R, Milsom I. A longitudinal population-based survey of urinary incontinence,

overactive bladder, and other lower urinary tract symptoms in women. Eur Urol. 2009;55:783–91.

3. Abrams P, Cardozo L, Khoury S, Wein A, editors. 3rd international consultation on incontinence. Annex 2: International Consultation on Incontinence Modular Questionnaire (ICIQ) UI SF (short form). London: Health Publications Ltd; 2005. p. 1630.

4. Abrams P, Cardozo L, Khoudry S, Wein A, editors. 3rd international consultation on incontinence. London: Health Publications Ltd; 2005. p. 1607.

5. Catalona WJ, Carvalhal GF, Mager DE, et al. Potency, continence and complication rates in 1,870 consecutive radical retropubic prostectomies. J Urol. 1999;162:433–8.

6. Eden CG, Moon DA. Laparoscopic radical prostatectomy: minimum 3-year follow-up of the first 100 patients in the UK. BJU Int. 2006;97:981–4.

Chapter 10
Recurrent Urinary Tract Infections in Adults

Rhana Hassan Zakri and M. Shamim Khan

Definitions [1]

Cystitis

Clinical constellation of symptoms causing dysuria on voiding, urinary frequency and urgency often associated with suprapubic pain.

Urinary Tract Infection (UTI)

UTI is defined as an inflammatory response of the urothelium to microbial invasion. Traditionally this has been quantitatively defined by the presence of $>10^5$ bacteria/ml of urine. However, 20–40 % of women may be symptomatic at lower bacterial counts. On the contrary contamination of urine in uncircumcised men may show a high count in otherwise

R.H. Zakri, MBBS, MRCS, MSc (✉)
Department of Urology, Frimley Park Hospital, Frimley, UK
e-mail: rhzakri@doctors.org.uk

M. Shamim Khan, MBBS, MCPS, FRCS (Urol), FEBU
Department of Urology, Guy's and St. Thomas' NHS Foundation Trust, London, UK

B. Challacombe, S. Bott (eds.), *Diagnostic Techniques in Urology*, 87
DOI 10.1007/978-1-4471-2766-6_10,
© Springer-Verlag London 2014

asymptomatic males. Precedence is therefore now given to the presence or absence of cystitis symptoms rather than any strict criteria alone.

Bacteriuria

Is the presence of bacteria in the urine. Bacteriuria may be symptomatic or asymptomatic. This is indicated on a urine dip test by positive nitrites (Sensitivity 35–85 %, Specificity 92–100 %).

Pyuria

The presence of white blood cells (WBCs) in urine. Indicated on a urine dip test by positive leucocytes (Sensitivity 70–95 %).

Bacterial Colonization of Urine

The presence of bacteriuria without pyuria. This does not indicate active infection.

Recurrent Urinary Tract Infection

Two UTIs in the last 6 months or three in the last 12 months recurring after successful resolution of the previous episode.

Uncomplicated/Complicated UTI

An uncomplicated UTI is one occurring in a patient with a functionally and anatomically normal urinary tract without the presence of an underlying pathology known to increase the risk of infection. A complicated UTI occurs in a functionally or anatomically abnormal urinary tract or one with the following underlying risk factors (Table 10.1).

Table 10.1 Underlying risk factors for complicated UTIs

Functional/anatomical abnormality
Male gender
Elderly
Pregnancy
Indwelling catheter/stent/nephrostomy
Recurrent instrumentation
Diabetes
Immuno-suppression
Renal transplant
Renal failure
Recent hospital admission

Recurrent Urinary Tract Infection in Females [1–4]

Thirty to fifty percent of all women will suffer at least one UTI in their lifetime. Of these, 34–40 % will face significant ongoing morbidity at the hands of recurrent infections.

Figure 10.1 shows a pathway for initial patient work-up. It is important to tailor your assessment to the patient's age and establish early whether you are dealing with a likely complicated or uncomplicated UTI. Urinary tract tuberculosis in certain ethnic populations should also be kept in mind and therefore history of recent travel also enquired about.

Ascertain past medical history and surgical history. Enquire about current regular medications and whether the patient has had pelvic radiotherapy in the past. This will highlight the possibility of non-infective cystitis (Radiation/drug induced cystitis). Ask relevant sexual and menstrual history in conjunction with timing of UTIs.

Perform a full abdominal examination to look for previous operation scars, a palpable bladder, ballottable kidneys and

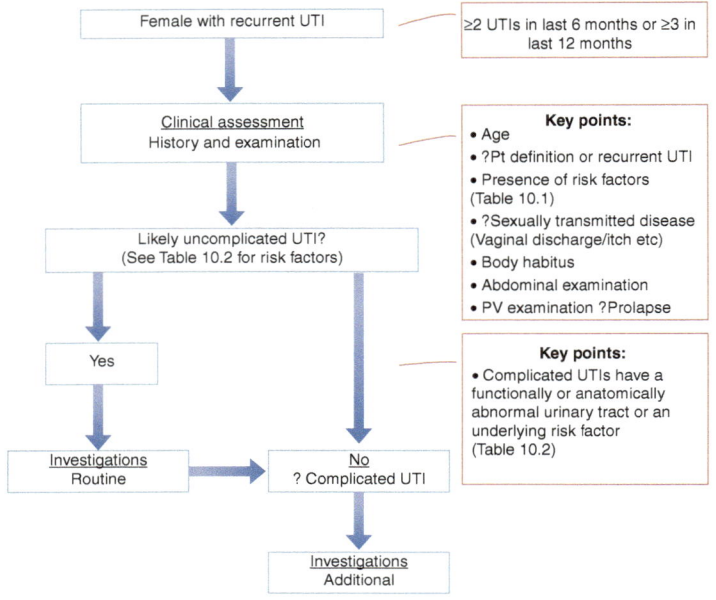

FIGURE 10.1 Initial assessment in females with recurrent UTI

elicit loin/supra-pubic tenderness. In the presence of a chaperone, perform a vaginal (PV) examination if you are comfortable doing so. Look for the presence of a tight urethral meatus, if visible, or a prolapse.

Figure 10.2 highlights the initial routine investigations to be performed in most cases of recurrent UTIs. Again, choose relevant investigations in conjunction with your clinical assessment. The aim should be to ascertain whether the UTI is complicated or uncomplicated and to find reversible causative factors. All patients with cystitis (see Table 10.2) or proven infection should have their urine cultured. This is not only to highlight the causative organism but also provide a guide about antibiotic sensitivities. Serial urine cultures in recurrent UTIs provide important insight into whether there is bacterial persistence or re-infection (See Fig. 10.4).

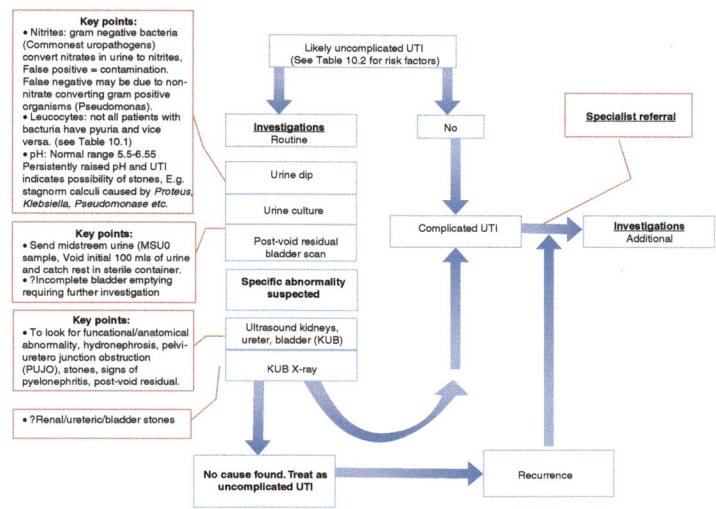

FIGURE 10.2 Investigating women with suspected uncomplicated recurrent UTIs

TABLE 10.2 Summary of definitions

Cystitis – Symptom constellation of dysuria, frequency, urgency +/− suprapubic pain

UTI – Urothelium's inflammatory response to microbial invasion

Bacteriuria – Presence of bacteria in urine

Pyuria – Presence of WBCs in urine

Colonization of urine – Presence of bacteriuria without pyuria

Recurrent UTIs – 2 UTIs in last 6 months or 3 in last 12 months recurring after resolution of previous episode

Complicated UTI – UTI in a functionally or anatomically abnormal urinary tract or one with underlying risk factors

Appropriate collection of urine by the patient is vital for accurate assessment and subsequent management. Ensure your patients are provided with a labeled sterile 'white topped' container to collect the urine. They should be instructed to wash their hands and genitalia before collection. Instruct the patient to void the initial 100 ml of urine before catching the midstream in the container. Please ensure that if the urine cannot be handed in within the next hour or so, it is placed in a sealed plastic bag and placed in the fridge. Any urine kept for longer than 24 h, even in the fridge, should be discarded and a fresh sample sought. A urine sample that has been standing for a long duration without refrigeration would encourage bacteria to multiply and give false readings. This should therefore also be discarded (Figs. 10.3 and 10.4).

All patients with suspected complicated UTIs should be referred to a urologist for specialist evaluation.

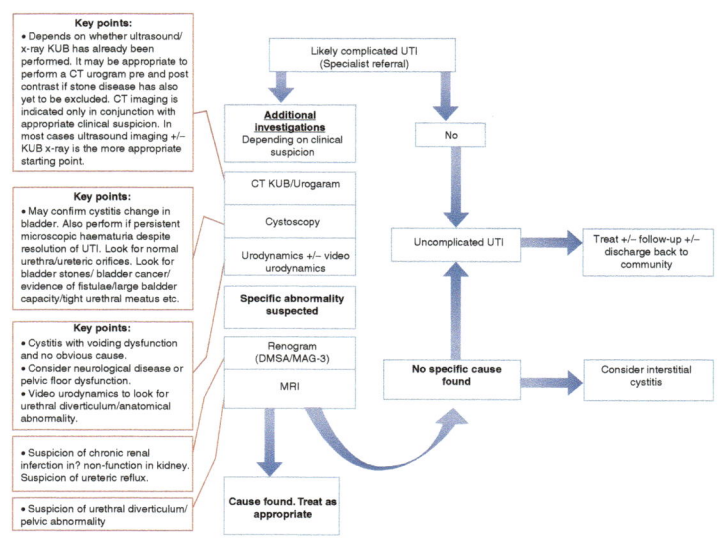

FIGURE 10.3 Investigating women with suspected complicated recurrent UTIs

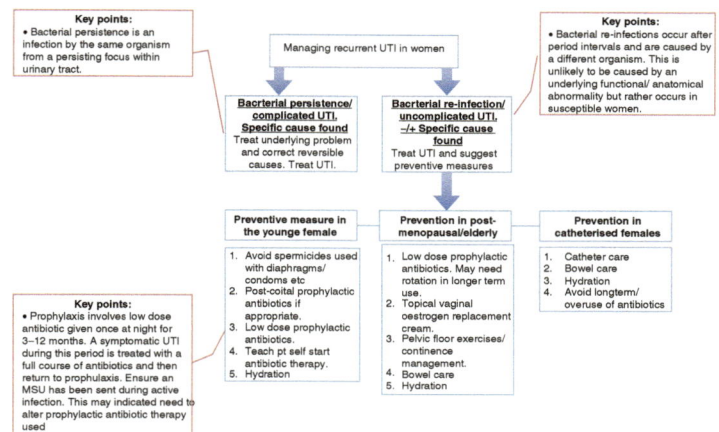

FIGURE 10.4 Management pathway for recurrent UTIs in women

TABLE 10.3 Summary of common Uropathogens

Bacteria	Infection
E-coli, Klebsiella, Staphylococcus, Proteus	Acute uncomplicated UTI
E-coli, Proteus, Klebsiella, Enterobacter, Staphylococcus	Acute uncomplicated pyelonephritis
E-coli, Enterobacter	Acute complicated UTI
Staphylococcus, Klebsiella, Proteus	Nosocomial UTI
Enterobacter, Pseudomonas, Candida	Acute complicated pyelonephritis
E-Coli, Klebsiella, Enterobacter, Proteus	Acute bacterial prostatitis (Men)

Please note that the algorithms above provide a broad overview of management. It is important that each pathway be considered in conjunction with patient specific factors in mind.

The table below shows the most common pathogens causing UTIs. Refer to your local hospital/community policy for antibiotic treatment (Table 10.3).

Recurrent Urinary Tract Infection in Men [5, 6]

Although recurrent UTIs in men are uncommon, it is thought that approximately 20 % of all UTIs occur in the male population. Of these only 0.1 % occur in men <50 years. The generally lower incidence of UTIs in men can be attributed to the following factors:

(a) Longer male urethra
(b) Antibacterial activity of prostate secretions
(c) Greater urethro-anal distance
(d) Less moisture around urethral meatus

Table 10.4 highlights some of the common causes of recurrent UTIs in men.

Figure 10.5 below gives an overview into the management of recurrent UTI in men. Please note that the management pathway should be tailored to the patient's age and likely causative factors as in the table above.

From the history elicit whether the patient is suffering from storage (frequency, nocturia, urgency, urgency incontinence) or voiding (hesitancy, poor stream, intermittency) lower urinary tract symptoms (LUTS). Ask whether their flow rate changed over a long duration or more acutely if at all. Enquire about painful ejaculation and the colour of the

TABLE 10.4 Risk factors for recurrent UTI in men

Young men (aged 18–35 years)	Older men >50 years
Phimosis	Bladder outlet obstruction (BPH)
Urethral strictures	Urinary retention Iatrogenic/instrumentation (i.e. TRUS prostate biopsies)
Stone disease	Cognitive impairment
Anal intercourse	Catheterisation
Sexually transmitted disease	Faecal/urinary incontinence
	Anal intercourse
	Previous urological surgery

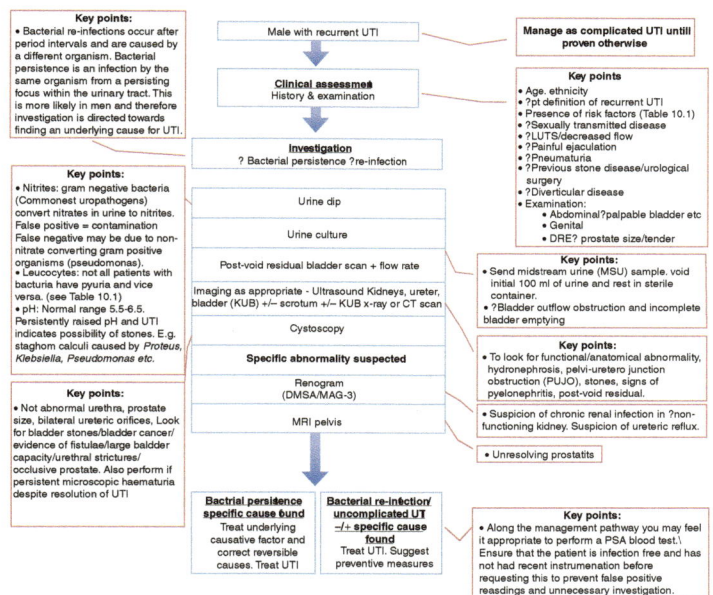

Key points:
• Bacterial re-infections occur after period intervals and are caused by a different organism. Bacterial persistence is an infection by the same organism from a persisting focus within the urinary tract. This is more likely in men and therefore investigation is directed towards finding an underlying cause for UTI.

Male with recurrent UTI

Manage as complicated UTI untill proven otherwise

Key points
• Age, ethnicity
• ?pt definition of recurrent UTI
• Presence of risk factors (Table 10.1)
• ?Sexually transmitted disease
• ?LUTS/decreased flow
• ?Painful ejaculation
• ?Pneumaturia
• ?Previous stone disease/urological surgery
• ?Diverticular disease
• Examination:
   • Abdominal?palpable bladder etc
   • Genital
   • DRE? prostate size/tender

Clinical assessment
History & examination

Investigation
? Bacterial persistence ?re-infection

Key points:
• Nitrites: gram negative bacteria (Commonest uropathogens) convert nitrates in urine to nitrites. False positive = contamination False negative may be due to non-nitrate converting gram positive organisms (pseudomonas).
• Leucocytes: not all patients with bacturia have pyuria and vice versa. (see Table 10.1)
• pH: Normal range 5.5-6.5. Persistently raised pH and UTI indicates possibility of stones. E.g. staghorn calculi caused by *Proteus, Klebsiella, Pseudomonas* etc.

Urine dip

Urine culture

Post-void residual bladder scan + flow rate

Key points:
• Send midstream urine (MSU) sample. void initial 100 ml of urine and rest in sterile container.
• ?Bladder outflow obstruction and incomplete bladder emptying

Imaging as appropriate - Ultrasound Kidneys, ureter, bladder (KUB) +/– scrotum +/– KUB x-ray or CT scan

Cystoscopy

Key points:
• To look for functional/anatomical abnormality, hydronephrosis, pelvi-uretero junction obstruction (PUJO), stones, signs of pyelonephritis, post-void residual.

Specific abnormality suspected

Key points:
• Not abnormal urethra, prostate size, bilateral ureteric orifices. Look for bladder stones/bladder cancer/ evidence of fistulae/large baldder capacity/urethral strictures/ occlusive prostate. Also perform if persistent microscopic haematuria despite resolution of UTI

Renogram
(DMSA/MAG-3)

MRI pelvis

• Suspicion of chronic renal infection in ?non-functioning kidney. Suspicion of ureteric reflux.

• Unresolving prostatits

Bactrial persistence specific cause found
Treat underlying causative factor and correct reversible causes. Treat UTI

Bacterial re-infection/ uncomplicated UT –/+ specific cause found
Treat UTI. Suggest preventive measures

Key points:
• Along the management pathway you may feel it appropriate to perform a PSA blood test.\ Ensure that the patient is infection free and has not had recent instrumentation before requesting this to prevent false positive readings and unnecessary investigation.

FIGURE 10.5 Management pathway for recurrent UTIs in men

ejaculate. Pain in the perineal region, particularly on sitting down may indicate prostatitis and should therefore be investigated as such if a digital rectal examination (DRE) supports this diagnosis (Tender prostate that may feel boggy). Prostatitis is one indication where it is appropriate to send a PSA blood test during infection. This allows diagnostic confirmation and also shows improvement with resolution after treatment. In patients with a past history of diverticular disease/diverticulitis, ask about the presence of pneumaturia to rule out colovesical fistula. Perform a full abdominal examination that includes the genitalia and DRE. Look for evidence of an infected hydrocele/epididymo-orchitis that may require further investigation and treatment.

Discussing the management of individual causative factors is beyond the remit of this chapter. Please refer to the appropriate chapters for such information.

TABLE 10.5 Prevalence of antibiotic resistance to common uropathogens [7–9]

Uropathogen	Prevalence of resistance (approximate %)					
	Trimeth	Nitro	Amox	Cipro	Co-amox	Gent
E-Coli	34	12	52	24	10	12
Proteus	55.6	22.2	4.5	–	1.0	–
Klebsiella	20	–	83.5	24	4.1	16
Coliforms	75	25	2.5	20.5	21.3	11.5
Pseudomonas	50	–	–	24	–	16.5

Key: *Trimeth* trimethoprim, *Nitro* nitrofurantoin, *Amox* amoxicillin, *Cipro* ciprofloxacin, *Co-amox* co-amoxiclav, *Gent* gentamicin

Please refer to Table 10.3 for common uropathogens. Whilst the literature suggests *E-coli* to be the most common uropathogen causing both hospital acquired and community based UTIs, studies have also shown a high Gram positive prevalence (47 and 28 % respectively of all out-patient UTI urine cultures), and in particular, *Enterococci* [1].

An acute symptomatic UTI with no signs of sepsis should be treated with a five-seven-day course of oral antibiotics. A common antibiotic choice is Trimethoprim but Amoxycillin has significant resistance. It should be kept in mind however, the importance of referring to local guidelines for antibiotic treatment policies. Patients should be encouraged to complete their antibiotic course even if symptoms resolve. This is to prevent antibiotic resistance as much as possible. Also, avoid over zealous use of antibiotics and ensure a rational approach to prescribing.

A study by DasGupta et al. in 2009 has shown as high as 30–40 % resistance of *E-Coli* to Trimethoprim and a 25 % resistance to Ciprofloxacin at their hospital. Local practice should therefore be evidence based according to local microbial prevalence and trends in antibiotic resistance. This should be reviewed on a regular basis. Table 10.5 shows an example of the prevalence of antibiotic resistance. It gives a good understanding into the better antibiotic choice for a particular organism cultured.

Table 10.5 above worryingly demonstrates how widespread use of Trimethoprim in the community for example, has led to rising levels of resistance by most common uro-pathogens. This table can be used as a guide into the antibiotic choices that you make. We must emphasis however, that this is a generalised table and that figures for your local area may vary.

Innovation in the Management of Recurrent UTIs: The Role of Vaccines

The ability of an organism to cause disease is known as virulence. It is characterized by both host and microbial factors. Of particular significance is bacterial uro-colonisation and host invasion by way of their ability to adhere irreversibly, (via bacterial fimbriae/P-pilli for example), to urothelium and cause infection. The discovery of antibodies that prevent adherence of bacteria to urothelial cells is being formulated in the form of a vaccine that hopes to revolutionize the preventative management of recurrent UTIs in the future. Refer to our article, 'Preventing recurrent urinary tract infections: role of vaccines' by Zakri RH et al. for more information [10].

References

1. Dason S, Dason J, Kapoor A, et al. Guidelines for the diagnosis and management of urinary tract infection in women. Can Urol Assoc J. 2001;5(5):316–22.
2. Dwyer P, O'Reilly M. Recurrent urinary tract infection in the female. Chapter urogynaecology. Curr Opin Obstet Gynaecol. 2002;14:537–43.
3. Hooten T. Recurrent urinary tract infection in women. Int J Antimicrob Agents. 2001;17:259–68.
4. Nosseir S, Lind L, Winkler H. Recurrent uncomplicated urinary tract infections in women: a review. J Womens Health (Larchmt). 2012;21(3):347–54.
5. Andrews SJ, Brooks PT, Hanbury DC, et al. Ultrasonography and abdominal radiography versus intravenous urography in investigation of urinary tract infection in men: prospective incident cohort study. BMJ. 2002;324:454–6.

6. Griebling TL. Urinary tract infection in men. Urologic Diseases in America. Litwin MS, Saigal CS. Washington, DC, US Department of Health and Human Services, Public Health Service, National Institutes of Health, National Institute of Diabetes and Digestive and Kidney Diseases; US Government Printing Office. http://kidney.niddk.nih.gov/statistics/uda/. 2007, 623–45.

7. DasGupta R, Sullivan R, French G, et al. Evidence based prescription of antibiotics in urology: a 5 year review of microbiology. BJU Int. 2009;104:760–4.

8. Ipek I, Bozaykut A, Caktir D, et al. Antimicrobial resistance patterns of uropathogens among children in Istanbul, Turkey. Southeast Asian J Trop Med Public Health. 2011;42(2): 355–62.

9. Kahlmeter G. An international survey of the antimicrobial susceptibility of pathogens from uncomplicated urinary tract infections: the ECO SENS Project. J Antimicrob Chemother. 2003;51:69–76.

10. Zakri RH, DasGupta R, Dasgupta P, et al. Preventing recurrent urinary tract infections: role of vaccines. BJU Int. 2008;102: 1055–6.

Chapter 11
Loin Pain

Timothy Nedas and Matthew Bultitude

The loin describes the posterior-lateral extent of the abdomen inferior to the twelfth rib, superior to the pelvis and lateral to the sacrospinous ligament. The loin generally does not include the midline posterior lumbar region. Pain in the loin has multiple differential diagnoses, which can be filtered with history, examination and simple practice-based diagnostic tests to give a diagnosis.

From a urological perspective one can initially classify the differentials of loin pain as urological and non-urological. These are summarised in Table 11.1.

History

Loin pain may be acute or present more insidiously. The pain may be constant or occur in waves. The intensity can vary from mild discomfort to severe pain.

T. Nedas, MBBS, Msc, FRCS (Urol)
Department of Urology,
Guy's and St. Thomas' Hospitals NHS Foundation Trust,
London, UK

M. Bultitude, MBBS, MRCS, MSc, FRCS (Urol) (✉)
Department of Urology,
Guy's and St. Thomas' NHS Foundation Trust, London, UK
e-mail: matthew.bultitude@gsttt.nhs.uk

B. Challacombe, S. Bott (eds.), *Diagnostic Techniques in Urology*, 99
DOI 10.1007/978-1-4471-2766-6_11,
© Springer-Verlag London 2014

TABLE 11.1 Differential diagnoses of loin pain

Urological causes	Non urological causes
Urinary Tract Infection (UTI)	Musculoskeletal injury
Pyelonephritis	Aortic aneurysm or dissection
Renal calculi	Nerve root pain
Infected obstructed kidney	Appendicitis
Extrinsic compression of ureter by retroperitoneal mass	Diverticulitis
Pelviureteric junction obstruction	Cholecystits
	Gynecological pain
	Lower zone pneumonia/pleritis

Assessment

It is vital to take a full history in all patients presenting with loin pain (see below). This will often help guide further investigations based on the likely clinical cause. Pulse, blood pressure and temperature should be documented. A full abdominal examination should be performed. This should include examination of the external genitalia in men (as testicular pathology may present with abdominal pain) and a bimanual vaginal examination in women. Examination of the abdomen should localise the area of pain and report any focal or generalised tenderness, guarding or rebound. If musculoskeletal cause is suspected then an assessment of the back should be made for bony or muscular tenderness. Is the pain reproduced by movement of the spine or straight leg raise? It may be appropriate to examine for lower limb neurology.

Investigation begins with urinalysis. Nitrites are strongly predictive of the presence of infection, whilst other positive findings can represent both urological and peritoneal problems. Table 11.2 summarises the indications for hospital referral.

If the patient is not being referred then outpatient imaging may be required. An ultrasound scan is useful for eliminating

TABLE 11.2 Indications for hospital admission with suspected renal colic

Indications for acute hospital admission
Diagnostic uncertainty (consider admission for patients older than 60 years, because a leaking aortic aneurysm could present with similar symptoms)
Inability to obtain or maintain adequate pain control
Presence of significant fever (>37.5 °C) in association with suspected renal colic
Renal colic in patient with solitary or transplanted kidney
Suspected bilateral obstructing stones
Impending acute renal failure
Inability to arrange early investigation or urological assessment

hydronephrosis and can examine the gall bladder and gynecological organs. However it may not be reliable for assessing urological stone disease, although the sensitivity can be improved by obtaining a plain abdominal film. If stone disease is suspected a non contrast CT scan is the gold-standard investigation as this will identify virtually all calculi (other than very rare matrix or indinavir stones) and may also pick up other abdominal pathology [1, 2]. An intravenous urogram is less favoured as the radiological investigation of choice in stone disease.

Acute Loin Pain

If one suspects a leaking aortic aneurysm or aortic dissection then immediate emergency referral to the local vascular service is advised. The age (over 60), sex (male), a previous history of vascular disease and information about the smoking habits of the patient should allow a rapid inclusion or exclusion of aortic pathology

Acute sudden onset loin pain associated with strenuous exercise and a specific strain is likely to be due to muscle injury and should initially be managed with analgesia. Similarly acute pain in the flank following trauma may be a rib fracture although it may also represent renal trauma. Acceleration/deceleration injuries or direct force to the flank may result in damage to the renal pedicle or a renal haematoma. A urine dipstick positive for microscopic haematuria or indeed frank haematuria are significant findings. All adults with frank haematuria and all children with frank or microscopic haematuria following trauma should have imaging of their urinary tract. (EAU guidelines) [1].

Acute relapsing, remitting pain in the loin, which may radiate to the groin and testicles or labia, may well be renal colic due to stone obstruction. A previous history of stone disease is clearly a risk factor as are diabetes, obesity and an occupation involving a hot environment. The patient should be assessed for signs of sepsis and if present urgent urological referral arranged. Visible haematuria in this situation may be a feature of colic due to stone disease but it could also represent bleeding due to other pathology in the urinary tract.

Acute relapsing remitting pain that radiates to the right upper quadrant rather than to the groin may be cholecystitis especially if the pain is associated with eating. Whilst an abdominal ultrasound may show calcified gallstones and may show renal calculi, a non contrast CT-KUB (the current secondary care gold standard for urinary tract calculi) will probably not reveal the presence of gallstones.

Acute constant pain in the loin can represent intraperitoneal causes of pain; on the right hand side appendicitis should be considered particularly if the patient is additionally tender over the right iliac fossa and McBurney's point. Similar pain but on the left may well be due to diverticulitis. In females such pain may be due to ruptured ovarian cysts or an ectopic pregnancy. A patient that shows signs of peritonism on examination (guarding and rebound) is more likely to have a non urological cause for their symptoms than urological, even in the presence of microscopic haematuria.

Acute constant loin pain with a fever and often accompanied by dysuria, frequency, urgency or other symptoms of urinary tract infection may represent pyelonephritis. In this situation it is important to examine the urine with both a dipstick test and mid stream urine (by definition a urinary tract infection ascending to the kidney is not a simple infection and therefore an MSU should be sent). If the patient shows signs of sepsis then urgent imaging to exclude infection resulting from urinary tract obstruction should be arranged, this is also the case if one suspects sepsis from the urinary tract without symptoms of UTI. If the patient is not septic then imaging should be carried out but this may be done on a semi-urgent (within a few days) basis. Patients who have had pyelonephritis will continue to experience pain for some weeks after the infection has been successfully treated.

Pregnancy can cause loin pain and this can be hard to interpret particularly as all women will develop some degree of hydronephrosis (the right is usually more affected than the left). Women who have been pregnant more than once or had previous urological disease can often distinguish between loin pain of pregnancy and loin pain of another cause. Pregnant women with significant loin pain should have an ultrasound scan in addition to a urine dipstick and MSU.

Rarer Cases

Patients with chronic debilitating diseases may be prone to forming renal calculi and it may be hard to interpret a mild loin ache and slight decrease in their general function as anything untoward. However it would be worth arranging imaging to exclude incipient obstruction as a cause of their symptoms.

Patients known to have polycystic kidney disease may experience acute pain when a cyst bleeds or ruptures. This can often present with visible haematuria and significant pain. These patients generally require hospital assessment to manage their pain as well as ensuring that they do not get urinary retention from clots.

Sickle cell disease and diabetes mellitus can cause papillary necrosis and sloughed papilla can cause acute pain that mimics renal colic from stone disease.

Chronic Loin Pain

Non Urological

Given the proximity of the spine and nerve roots to the loin chronic loin pain can have multiple causes. The patient's history may point to previous injury or shingles as a cause.

Urological

Renal calculi can cause chronic loin pain although it can often be hard to distinguish between incidental calculi and other causes of pain, in this circumstance stone treatment may be undertaken to help either cure pain or eliminate renal calculi as a cause. Parenchymal rather than collecting system calcification may also be a cause for pain [3]. Any tumour arising from the kidney may cause pain although small (less than 4 cm) renal masses and cysts do not tend to cause pain. Pelvi-ureteric junction obstruction can be a cause of chronic pain in all age groups and the pain is often exacerbated by a fluid load due to further distension of the renal pelvis. Previous renal surgery (open, minimally invasive or percutaneous) may cause chronic loin pain. Urologists often stent the urinary tract post operatively and these stents can cause pain whilst still in place.

Rarer urological causes of chronic loin pain include reflux disease, loin pain haematuria syndrome, retroperitoneal fibrosis and renal ptosis. Reflux disease causes pain when urine travels up to the kidney during bladder contraction, it normally occurs if the ureter does not have a normal insertion into the bladder (a long intramural portion of ureter usually prevents urinary reflux); it can also be caused by the presence of a ureteric stent. Loin pain haematuria syndrome is a relatively poorly understood condition that afflicts patients to varying degrees. It's name describes its symptoms accurately and it is a diagnosis reached when all other causes of loin pain and haematuria have been excluded, management is usually symptomatic and may involve referral to a pain specialist. Retroperitoneal fibrosis or tumour resulting in extrinsic ureteric obstruction may cause pain however often the obstruction is insipid and painless.

Conclusion

The assessment of loin pain requires attention to the core clinical skills of history and examination in conjunction with simple bedside tests (observations and urinalysis). Whilst "Common things are common" it is important to ensure that rare serious causes such as a leaking abdominal aortic aneurysm are excluded. In the majority this can be done clinically but beware the older patient, especially if they have no previous history of stone disease. Usually a non contrast CT scan will prove the diagnosis. The other key consideration is infection and any suspected urinary tract obstruction with suggestion of sepsis requires urgent assessment.

References

1. Turk C, et al. European Association of Urology guidelines on urolithiasis. 2012 http://www.uroweb.org/gls/pdf/20_Urolithiasis_LR%20March%2013%202012.pdf.
2. British Association of Urological Surgeons Guidelines for Acute management of first presentation of renal/ureteric lithiasis (excluding pregnancy). Updated Feb 2012 http://www.baus.org.uk/Resources/BAUS/Documents/PDF%20Documents/Sections/Endourology/Revised%20Acute%20Stone%20Mgt%20Guidelines.pdf.
3. Bultitude M, Rees J. Management of renal colic. BMJ. 2012; 345:e5499. doi:10.1136/bmj.e5499.

Chapter 12
Recurrent Stone Formers

Azhar Khan and Matthew Bultitude

The lifetime risk of forming a kidney stone among Caucasian men is about 8–10 %, and the peak incidence of stones occurs between the ages of 20–50 years. Among patients who have formed one kidney stone, the lifetime recurrence rate is 60–80 % while 10 % of men will form another stone within a year. There is significant geographic and seasonal variation in rates of stone recurrence. Genetic, environmental and metabolic factors are implicated in the pathogenesis of stone formation [1]. Therefore, specific metabolic evaluation of recurrent stone formers might identify risk factors [2], leading to proper medical and dietary therapies to prevent stone formation [3]. The evaluation of patients with nephrolithiasis consists of radiographic imaging along with blood and urine testing. There is a general agreement that a complete and specific metabolic evaluation is indicated in all patients with recurrent stone formation but it is not cost-effective for patients who have formed only one stone [4].

A. Khan, MBBS, MRCS
M. Bultitude, MBBS, MRCS, MSc, FRCS (Urol) (✉)
Department of Urology, Guy's and St. Thomas'
NHS Foundation Trust, London, UK
e-mail: matthew.bultitude@gsttt.nhs.uk

B. Challacombe, S. Bott (eds.), *Diagnostic Techniques in Urology*,   107
DOI 10.1007/978-1-4471-2766-6_12,
© Springer-Verlag London 2014

Presentation and Risk Factors

Most patients with renal stone disease present with acute renal colic or flank pain but some may present with haematuria or recurrent UTIs and others may be asymptomatic. As all recurrent stone-formers begin as single stone formers, it is important to assess the risk factors for stone recurrence in all patients with urinary stone disease. Every patient should be assigned to either a low-risk or high-risk group of stone formers [4]. This will allow for earlier recognition of any abnormality and may assist in the prevention of recurrent stone formation. Factors that put patients in the high risk category for subsequent stone formation include

- Multiple stones on imaging
- Young age at presentation
- Family history of stones
- Previous history of a stone
- GI diseases e.g. Bowel resection, Inflammatory bowel disease
- Gout/Uric acid stones
- Chronic UTIs
- Hyperparathyroidism
- Anatomical factors

  – Medullary Sponge kidney
  – Horseshoe kidney
  – Calyceal Diverticulum

- Genetic factors

  – Cystinuria
  – Renal tubular acidosis (RTA)
  – Primary Hyperoxaluria

Evaluation and Investigations

The initial evaluation of a patient with recurrent stones includes a thorough urological history with a particular focus on risk factors and a detailed description of previous stone events. Previous stone analyses should be sought. Serum calcium, uric acid and creatinine are usually checked as a first line investigation to exclude significant abnormalities in renal function and calcium/uric acid metabolism. Serum phosphate does not appear to be an independent risk factor for urinary tract stone recurrence or complications, nor is it a reliable early predictor of occult disease. An algorithm of a management protocol is shown in the algorithm (Fig. 12.1).

Urinalysis

A routine urinalysis provides useful information and cultures should be obtained when indicated. Persistent elevation of the fasting urinary pH over 5.8 suggests a degree of renal tubular acidosis (RTA). Urine microscopy of fresh urine may also identify crystalline elements that point to a diagnosis, for example, cystine crystals.

Radiological Imaging

CT KUB has become the gold standard investigation for renal stone disease and helps to assess stone burden as well as anatomical abnormalities such as horse-shoe kidney, calyceal diverticula or medullary sponge kidney.

Stone Analysis

Chemical analysis of a calculus passed in the urine or removed surgically is very helpful in elucidating the underlying cause and is recommended in all stone formers [4]. It is a good starting point for the metabolic evaluation and can also help determine if further investigation will be worthwhile. Thus patients should be encouraged to retain any stone passed in their urine.

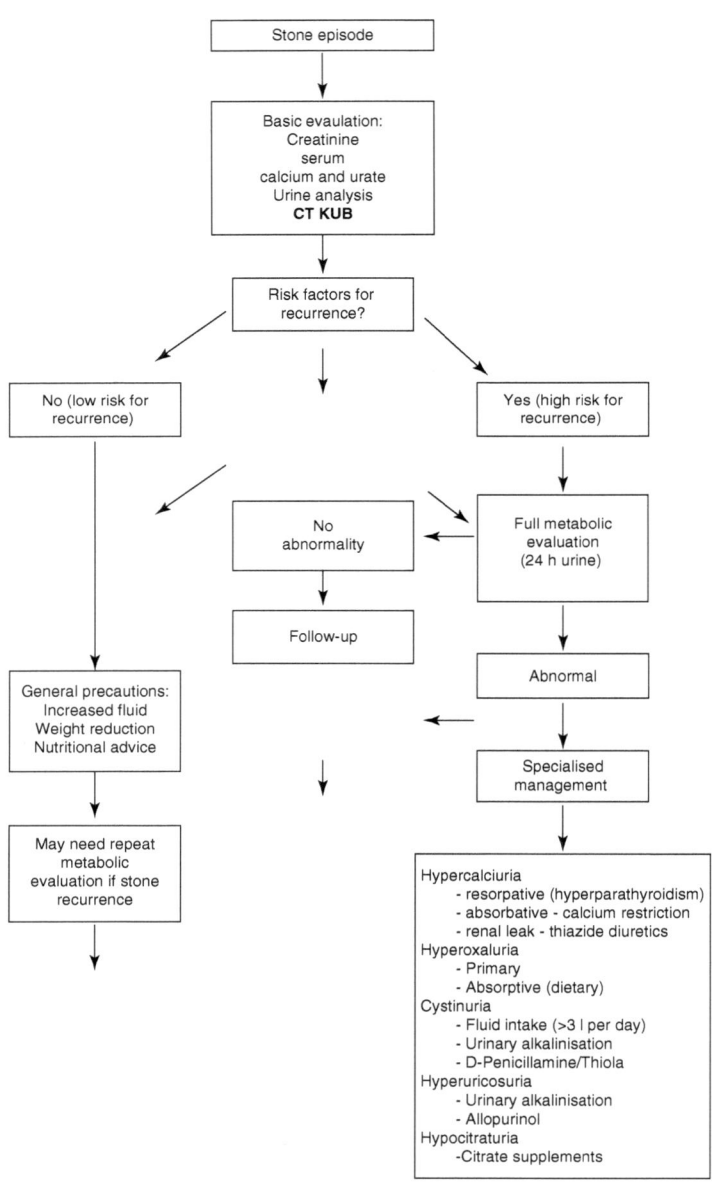

FIGURE 12.1 Management algorithm for recurrent stone disease

Urinary Metabolic Assessment

In the assessment of patients with recurrent urinary stone disease, 24 h urine collections give important information on the risk of recurrent stone formation. A minimum of 20 days is recommended between stone expulsion or surgical removal and 24-h urine collection to allow patients to return to their normal habits [5]. If performed earlier, urine volumes will be inappropriately high and urinary excretion of calcium inappropriately low and therefore the risk of recurrent stone formation is underestimated. Specific metabolic evaluation generally requires the collection of two consecutive 24-h urine samples, one in a bottle with hydrochloric acid for calcium, oxalate, phosphate, cystine, citrate and magnesium, and one in a plain bottle to measure uric acid, pH and electrolytes. The most common findings on 24 h urine studies include hypercalciuria, hyperoxaluria, hyperuricosuria, hypocitraturia, and low urinary volume.

Urinary pH

Patients with a fixed low urinary pH tend to produce uric acid crystals because of the low solubility of uric acid in an acidic environment. In addition to dietary moderation of animal protein intake, either potassium citrate or sodium bicarbonate can be used to alkalinise the urine. Potassium citrate may be preferred in stone formers to avoid the salt load (and in patients with cystinuria, where sodium bicarbonate can cause a rise in cystine excretion). While taking either of these drugs, patients should frequently monitor their urinary pH.

The most common causes of a high urinary pH are urinary tract infection with a urea-splitting micro-organisms and renal tubular acidosis (RTA). Persistently elevated urinary pH values above 7.2 are associated with an increased precipitation of calcium phosphate crystals either alone or as calcium magnesium ammonium phosphate (infection stone).

Management

Although in some cases renal stone disease is the consequence of specific hereditary or acquired diseases, the most common form is idiopathic calcium nephrolithias (calcium oxalate stones) resulting from supersaturation of calcium oxalate and/or calcium phosphate. Fluid intake, dietary habits and lifestyle have a direct effect on the pathogenesis of these stones. Irrespective of the patient risk group these factors can be modified as first line and therefore will have a direct impact on the stone recurrence rate (Fig. 12.1).

Role of Fluid Intake

Low 24-h urine volume indicates poor fluid intake. Good fluid intake is the single most important factor that should be advised at every possible opportunity. All patients with recurrent stones should strive to achieve a urine output of more than 2 L daily as this has been shown in a randomised trial to significantly reduce stone episodes [6]. In this study, participants were randomized to >2 l/day of water intake versus no treatment for 5 years. Those with high water intake had significantly less stone recurrence rate (12 % vs. 27 %, $p = 0.008$). In addition, large epidemiologic studies have shown high urinary volume as an effective way of stone prevention in the general population. Patients with cystine stones or those with resistant cases may need a daily urinary output of 3 L and may need to wake at night to drink. With urine output less than 1 L/day, even the urine of a normal subject reaches extremely high supersaturation levels. An increase in fluids is, therefore, efficacious because it reduces the relapse rate and increases the time to relapse.

Dietary Modifications

Depending on the cause of the kidney stones, dietary changes are sometimes recommended to decrease the likelihood of developing further kidney stones. A restriction in dietary calcium is not advisable as a low-calcium diet does not reduce urinary calcium levels, but instead increases the intestinal absorption of oxalate, which can increase the risk of stone recurrence. In one study, the relapse rate was significantly lower in patients on a normal-calcium, low-protein, low-salt diet than in patients on a low-calcium diet [7]. High protein diet especially from an animal source can cause hyperuricosuria because of an increase in the intake and endogenous production of purines, and therefore increases the risk of uric acid stone formation. Fruits and vegetables are not only a source of extra fluid but also provide citrate, which is an important chelating agent for calcium. Ascorbic acid (Vitamin C supplementation) is an oxalate precursor, and therefore, excessive intake is to be discouraged in subjects with kidney stones.

Obesity and Weight Gain

Patients should be encouraged to weight control. Obesity, insulin resistance, metabolic syndrome, and diabetes have been associated with kidney stones, particularly those caused by uric acid [8]. Excessive weight can cause insulin resistance and a compensatory hyperinsulinemia which in turn may contribute to the development of calcium stones by increasing the urinary excretion of calcium. Larger body size may also result in increased urinary excretion of uric acid and oxalate, risk factors for calcium oxalate kidney stones.

Metabolic Abnormalities

Patients in the high risk group for recurrent stone disease will need metabolic assessment. Common metabolic abnormalities are: hypercalciuria; hyperoxaluria; hyperuricosuria; cystinuria; renal tubular acidosis; hypercitraturia.

Hypercalciuria is the most common biochemical abnormality in the 24-h urine analysis usually associated calcium oxalate and phosphate stone disease. Hypercalciuria is subdivided into absorptive, resorptive, and renal categories.

Resorptive hypercalciuria is secondary to primary hyperparathyroidism and is usually associated with high serum calcium level. The other two forms can be differentiated by the response to a low calcium diet as well as to calcium loading. The distinction between these two forms may be considered relevant as the absorptive hypercalciuria can be controlled by moderate dietary calcium restriction, whereas the renal hypercalciuria is managed by a thiazide diuretic.

Hyperoxaluria can be primary (congenital), absorptive (idiopathic) or enteric. Primary hyperoxaluria is a rare autosomal recessive defect of oxalate metabolism that causes excessive endogenous oxalate production. Enteric hyperoxaluria is due to malabsorption and is usually associated with chronic diarrhoeal syndromes. Thus, enteric hyperoxaluria is most amenable to treatment through dietary calcium supplementation. Calcium works as an oxalate binder, reducing oxalate absorption from the GI tract. Calcium citrate is the recommended supplement.

High uric acid (hyperuricosuria) can be associated with uric acid stones but can also predispose to the formation of calcium-containing calculi by providing a nidus of uric acid for calcium oxalate crystals to bind to. Treatment involves potassium citrate supplementation (to alkalinise the urine), allopurinol (to reduce uric acid levels), or both.

Cystinuria is an inherited error of defective transport of the amino acids cystine, ornithine, arginine and lysine across intestinal and renal tubular cell membranes. Cystine is poorly soluble and thus these patients form cystine stones with the peak incidence in the second or third decades of life. The cyanide-nitroprusside spot test is used to detect cystiuria although 24-hour urinary citrate levels may be measured to differentiate between homozygous and heterozygous cystinuria. The aim of the management is to increase the solubility of cystine in the urine by increasing fluid intake (>3 L/day), urinary alkalinisation by potassium citrate (pH 7.0–7.5) and using complexing agents to bind with cystine to make it more soluble such as D-penicillamine, thiola or captopril.

Renal tubular acidosis (RTA) is due to impaired secretion of H^+ in the distal renal tubule leading to poor acidification of urine (urinary pH never goes below 5.8). Hypercalciuria follows from bone resorption with recurrent stone formation. Confirmation of the diagnosis requires ammonium chloride loading test.

Citrate is an important chemical inhibitor of stone formation. Some studies have recommended citrate therapy as primary or adjunctive therapy to almost all patients who have formed recurrent calcium-containing stones. Potassium citrate is the preferred citrate supplement. Lemon juice or lemonade is an excellent alternate source of citrate with the added benefit of providing increased fluid intake.

Anatomical Abnormalities

Anatomical abnormalities with or without metabolic derangements pose a management challenge. Common abnormalities are Horseshoe kidney, calyceal diverticulum and medullary sponge kidney (MSK). These patients need regular follow up to recognise early recurrence and their management will largely be in the specialist centres.

In summary, urinary stones are a recurrent problem in the majority of patients. All stone formers, independent of their individual risk, should follow the preventive measures. The main focus of these is increasing fluid intake to maintain good urine volume, normalisation of dietary habits and weight control. A systematic approach can help to identify several risk factors and metabolic abnormalities relevant to particular types of stones. Timely identification and correction of these abnormalities can prevent stone recurrence and growth.

References

1. Shakhssalim N, Gilani KR, Parvin M, et al. An assessment of parathyroid hormone, calcitonin, 1,25 (OH)2 vitamin D3, estradiol and testosterone in men with active calcium stone disease and evaluation of its biochemical risk factors. Urol Res. 2011;39:1–7.
2. Yagisawa T, Chandhoke PS, Fan J. Comparison of comprehensive and limited metabolic evaluations in the treatment of patients with recurrent calcium urolithiasis. J Urol. 1999;161:1449–52.

3. Levy FL, Adams-Huet B, Pak CY. Ambulatory evaluation of nephrolithiasis: an update of a 1980 protocol. Am J Med. 1995; 98:50–9.
4. Turk C, et al. European Association of Urology guidelines on urolithiasis. 2012. http://www.uroweb.org/gls/pdf/20_Urolithiasis_LR%20March%2013%202012.pdf.
5. Shekarriz B, Stoller ML. Uric acid nephrolithiasis: current concepts and controversies. J Urol. 2002;168(4 Pt 1):1307–14.
6. Borghi L, Meschi T, Amato F, et al. Urinary volume, water and recurrences in idiopathic calcium nephrolithiasis: a 5-year randomized prospective study. J Urol. 1996;155:839–43.
7. Borghi L, Schianchi T, Meschi T, et al. Comparison of two diets for the prevention of recurrent stones in idiopathic hypercalciuria. N Engl J Med. 2002;346:77–84.
8. Taylor EN, Stampfer MJ, Curhan GC. Obesity, weight gain, and the risk of kidney stones. JAMA. 2005;293(4):455–62.

Chapter 13
Testicular Mass and Acute Testicular Pain

Paul K. Hegarty

Introduction

Assessment of the genitalia is part and parcel of abdominal examination. This is a necessary skill for general surgeons and urologists and for the paediatric equivalents. Developing this skill requires knowledge of the anatomy and repeated examination.

Testicular Mass

Males presenting with testicular mass ought to be seen urgently in clinic as testicular cancer can have a short doubling time. The patient is likely to be very concerned and thus deserves urgent expert attention. While the patient may have been in denial for some time, once the presence of a testicular mass is recognised anxiety may be overt. Channels of rapid access are required so that any health professional can refer cases within days of presentation.

P.K. Hegarty, FRCS (Urol)
Department of Urology,
Guy's and St. Thomas' NHS Foundation Trust,
London, UK
e-mail: paulhego@hotmail.com

B. Challacombe, S. Bott (eds.), *Diagnostic Techniques in Urology*, 117
DOI 10.1007/978-1-4471-2766-6_13,
© Springer-Verlag London 2014

History

How long the mass has been present may give an idea as to its behaviour. This may be useful in particular in the minority of men who routinely perform testicular self-examination (TSE). Testis cancer may be painless or have an ache. It may have been noticed following a trauma. History of undescended testicle is important as is history of scrotal/groin surgery as it may impact subsequent treatment.

Examination

The patient should be examined in a warm room. General physique is checked for signs of metastatic disease. Lymph nodes are examined in the neck, axillae and groins. The abdomen is examined for masses or enlarged viscera. The contralateral testis should be gently examined first for reasons of comparison and to attempt to put him at ease. All urologists should carry a torch to check for transillumination. The mass is felt and its relationship to the testicular and paratesticular structures delineated, if possible. He may need to examined lying and standing if inguinal hernia or varicocele is suspected. Once the mass is felt, confirm with the patient that this is the one of concern, as he may have been feeling something else. At this stage a competent clinician may be able to reach a diagnosis without recourse to confirmatory investigations, especially with benign lesions such as an epididymal cyst. A malignant tumour arises from the body of the testis itself rather than from the epididymis or tunica vaginalis.

Laboratory Investigations

If testis cancer has not been ruled out, serum tumour markers should be assayed (alpha fetoprotein, β-human chorionic gonadotrophin, lactate dehydrogenase) as well as full blood count and liver function tests. Normal tumour markers do not rule out a testis cancer.

Ultrasound

Ultrasound can help demonstrate the mass relative to the testis. It can differentiate solid from cystic lesions and colour Doppler may show the vascularity of the lesion, testis and cord. If testis cancer is suspected ultrasound can confirm the intratesticular mass, the size of the lesion and examine the contralateral testis for features such as microlithiasis that may indicate the need for contralateral biopsy at the time of radical orchidectomy. Ultrasound is also useful in the presence of a tense hydrocele where the testis is impalpable. In assessing a male with cryptorchidism, examination of the groins by an experienced clinician performs at least as well as ultrasound [1].

MR

Magnetic resonance is usually a second line investigation reserved for cases of inconclusive sonography [2]. MR has less operator dependence as ultrasound, and thus may be more reproducible. However ultrasound remains the more usual imaging modality.

CT

CT is usually reserved as a staging tool when the diagnosis is testis cancer. CT with oral and intravenous contrast is performed of thorax, abdomen and pelvis. This can be before or after orchidectomy. If not available prior to surgery a chest x-ray should be performed to rule out cannon-ball metastases which, unrecognised, could seriously impact the general anaesthetic.

Acute Testicular Pain

Acute testicular pain is a frequent cause of attendance to the emergency department. As testicular torsion is among the differential diagnoses, urgent assessment is mandatory. As stated above, assessment of the male genitalia is within the remit of general surgeons and urologists. Competence of dealing with the diagnosis and management should be within the training of both disciplines. If testicular torsion is not confidently ruled out then the patient must proceed for emergency exploration of the scrotum.

History

Time of onset should be noted as this impacts viability in cases of testicular torsion. Many males will have had similar episodes in the past that should not reassure to the absence of torsion. The pain of testicular torsion is usually intense enough to be associated with vomiting.

Examination

The patient with scrotal pain can be quite distressed and anxious, so it is important to assess him in as comfortable an environment as possible. After examining the abdomen the scrotum should be inspected, looking for scrotal skin changes and lie of the testis. Bilateral cremasteric reflexes should be performed though there is no specific clinical sign that rules out testicular torsion e.g. intact cremasteric reflex [3]. However the presence of a localised exquisitely tender area which is seen to be dark under stretched skin, on the upper pole of the testis "blue dot sign" is pathognomic of torsion of hydatid of Morgagni. However even in such cases, it can be argued that scrotal exploration and removal of the infarcted tissue may hasten resolution. At this stage if a clinical diagnosis of possible testicular torsion is made, then the patient is transferred emergency exploration, as further investigations may only delay expedient treatment. If there is doubt, then further investigations should be performed urgently. If these are not available then surgical exploration should supercede ([10]).

Urinalysis

This may give indication of urinary tract infection (epididymo-orchitis), or haematuria from ureteric colic with referred scrotal pain. Abnormal urinalysis may be seen with testis torsion so the findings should be integrated with the clinical findings.

Colour Flow Ultrasound Doppler

Grey scale ultrasound may show other causes of pain such as epididymo-orchitis, however colour Doppler is helpful in showing the blood flow to the testis. It is important to compare the flow on each side as there may still be some capsular flow in the presence of testicular torsion. Doppler ultrasound is operator-dependent. A multicentre study of 208 boys with testicular torsion had normal or increased blood flow in 24 % of cases [5]. Detailed examination of the spermatic cord may show the point of torsion more confidently. This technique has a sensitivity of 97.3 % and a specificity of 99 % [6, 5] and thus should be integrated into the technique of scanning the scrotum in the setting of acute pain.

Other Imaging Modalities

Contrast enhanced ultrasound, scintigraphy and contast enhanced MR may have higher sensitivities and specificities in assessing acute scrotal pain however access to them may be limited and ought not delay urgent scrotal exploration [4, 7, 8].

Scrotal Exploration

This can be considered the gold-standard investigation of acute scrotal pain. This is the modality used in assessing accuracy of other investigations. The side effects of such treatment are low in contradistinction from the side effects of delayed or missed treatment of testicular torsion [3]. In the presence of unilateral torsion there is controversy on whether contralateral orchidopexy ought to be performed, though most surgeons fix the other side, to protect against future torsion [9].

Conclusion

Patients with testicular mass or pain require urgent and emergent care respectively. History and examination may suffice in their assessment, but often adjuvant modalities are needed, again with appropriate haste. Investigations need to be integrated sensibly with the clinical assessment. Ease of access to assessment and treatment is fundamental to minimising the physical and psychological harm of such events.

References

1. Elder JS. Ultrasonography is unnecessary in evaluating boys with a nonpalpable testis. Pediatrics. 2002;110(4):748–51.
2. Parenti GC, Feletti F, Brandini F, Palmarini D, Zago S, Ginevra A, Campioni P, Mannella P. Imaging of the scrotum: role of MRI. Radiol Med. 2009;114(3):414–24 [Article in English, Italian].
3. Hegarty PK, Walsh E, Corcoran MO. Exploration of the acute scrotum: a retrospective analysis of 100 consecutive cases. Ir J Med Sc. 2001;170:181–2.
4. Tekgül S, Riedmiller H, Gerharz E, Hoebeke P, Kocvara R, Nijman R, Radmayr Chr, Stein R. EAU/ESPU Paediatric urology guidelines (ISBN 978-90-79754-96-0), available at their website: http://www.uroweb.org/guidelines/online-guidelines/. Accessed 15 July 2012.
5. Kalfa N, Veyrac C, Lopez M, Lopez C, Maurel A, Kaselas C, Sibai S, Arena F, Vaos G, Breaud J, Merrot T, Kalfa D, Khochman I, Mironescu A, Minaev S, Averous M, Galifer RB. Multicenter assessment of ultrasound of the spermatic cord in children with acute scrotum. J Urol. 2007;177(1):297–301.

6. Kalfa N, Veyrac C, Baud C, Couture A, Averous M, Galifer RB. Ultrasonography of the spermatic cord in children with testicular torsion: impact on the surgical strategy. J Urol. 2004; 172(4 Pt 2):1692–5.

7. Mäkelä E, Lahdes-Vasama T, Ryymin P, Kähärä V, Suvanto J, Kangasniemi M, Kaipia A. Magnetic resonance imaging of acute scrotum. Scand J Surg. 2011;100(3):196–201.

8. Valentino M, Bertolotto M, Derchi L, Bertaccini A, Pavlica P, Martorana G, Barozzi L. Role of contrast enhanced ultrasound in acute scrotal diseases. Eur Radiol. 2011;21(9):1831–40.

9. Rhodes HL, Corbett HJ, Horwood JF, Losty PD. Neonatal testicular torsion: a survey of current practice amongst paediatric surgeons and urologists in the United Kingdom and Ireland. J Pediatr Surg. 2011;46(11):2157–60.

10. Tekgül S. Acute scrotum in children. In: Tekgul S, Riedmiller H, Gerharz E, et al. Guidelines on paediatric urology. Arnhem, The Netherlands: European Association of Urology, European Society for Paediatric Urology; 2009 Mar. p. 12–8. http://www.uroweb.org/gls/pdf/19_Paediatric_Urology.pdf.

Chapter 14
Penile Curvature

Nigel Borley

Overview

The symptom of penile curvature is almost invariably due to Peyronie's disease (often with associated discomfort from the shaft of the penis around the site of curvature with erections and sometimes with flaccidy of the erectile tissue distal to the plaque).

Men may be worried they have penile cancer, which will present as a painless swelling, rather than how it affects erections.

The important differential diagnoses are congenital penile curvature, chordee associated with hypospadias or epispadias, and rupture of the penile suspensory ligament.

A history of trauma is often looked for, and if you press men hard enough, most can come out with one event or other. If they readily remember an event of trauma with pain, swelling or bruising and detumescence that may have been a fracture that is significant. Otherwise the cause is thought to

N. Borley, BM, MRCS, MS, FRCS (Urol)
Department of Urology, Chelsea and Westminster Hospital,
London, UK
e-mail: nigelborley@hotmail.com

B. Challacombe, S. Bott (eds.), *Diagnostic Techniques in Urology*, 125
DOI 10.1007/978-1-4471-2766-6_14,
© Springer-Verlag London 2014

be repeated micro-trauma and abnormal tissue reaction. If they have Dupuytren's contracture, it helps them understand the process.

The development of the plaque is associated with vascular risk factors, but there plaque may restrict distal blood flow, particularly if the is an "hour-glass" deformity.

A congenital curvature is due to differing lengths of the corporal cavernosal bodies, or relatively different length of the corpus spongiosum. Chordee associated with hypospadias will often have been previously corrected, but there may be some residual chordee or a minor degree that were not previously evident.

A man may only start to realise he has congenital curvature once he gets older and starts to (inevitably) compare himself with others. It may take even longer for him to see someone about it. Congenital curvature is smoothly curved, rather than Peyronie's disease which appears angled, or a cork-screw if the plaque affects two planes.

As a result of a hard downward "tug" on the erect penis, a crack might be heard, which may be one of the suspensory ligaments at the base tearing. There may be some bruising at the base. This may make the penis appear to be angled or bend to one side as it becomes unsupported at the base.

A lot of men can get used to the appearance, the key to deciding on any intervention is how intercourse is affected and is it still possible.

Congenital ventral curvature

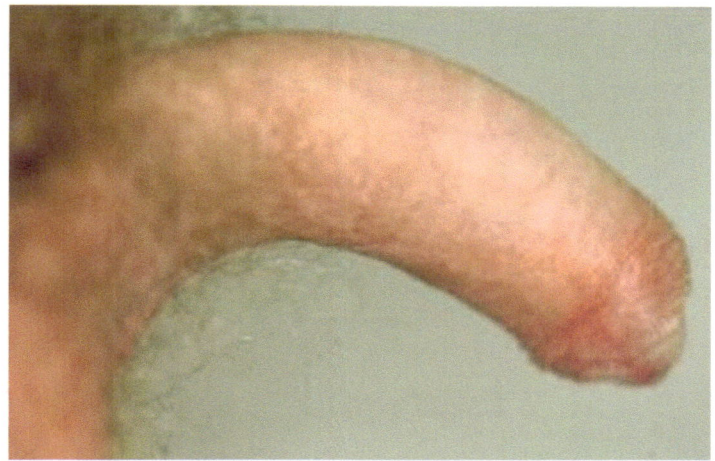

Congenital ventral curvature

Ventral curvature from Peyronie's plaque

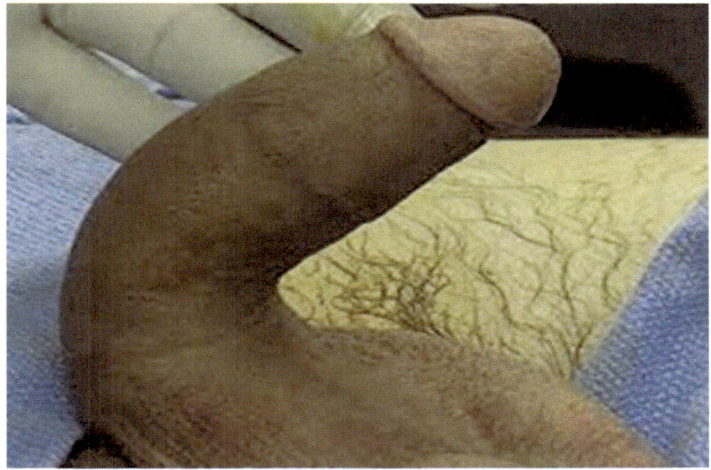

Ventral curvature from Peyronie's plaque

History – Duration

History –
Duration;

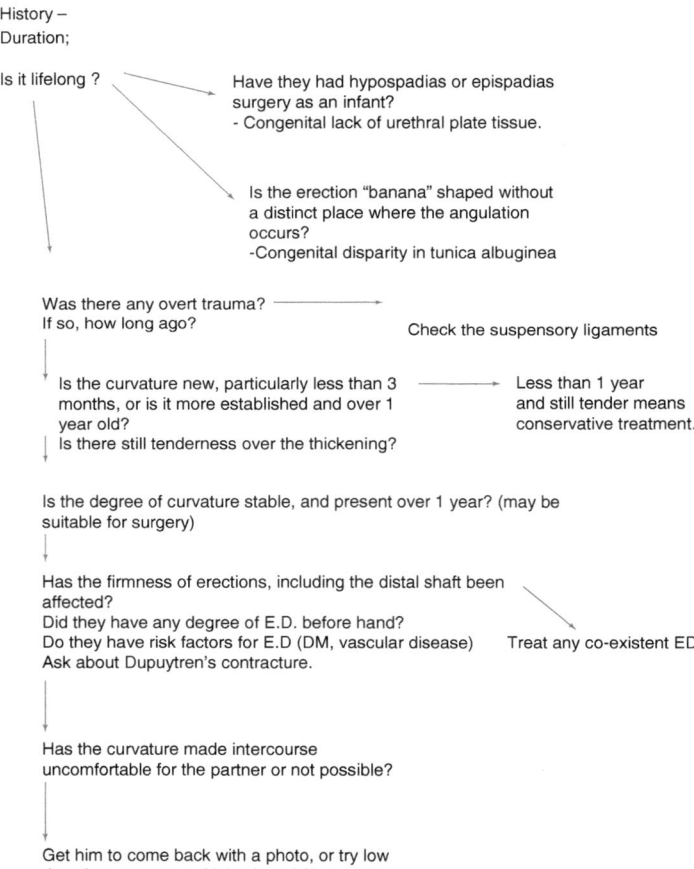

Is it lifelong ?

Have they had hypospadias or epispadias
surgery as an infant?
- Congenital lack of urethral plate tissue.

Is the erection "banana" shaped without
a distinct place where the angulation
occurs?
-Congenital disparity in tunica albuginea

Was there any overt trauma?
If so, how long ago?

Check the suspensory ligaments

Is the curvature new, particularly less than 3
months, or is it more established and over 1
year old?
Is there still tenderness over the thickening?

Less than 1 year
and still tender means
conservative treatment.

Is the degree of curvature stable, and present over 1 year? (may be
suitable for surgery)

Has the firmness of erections, including the distal shaft been
affected?
Did they have any degree of E.D. before hand?
Do they have risk factors for E.D (DM, vascular disease)
Ask about Dupuytren's contracture.

Treat any co-existent ED

Has the curvature made intercourse
uncomfortable for the partner or not possible?

Get him to come back with a photo, or try low
dose intra-cavernosal injection of Alprostadil

Examination

Palpate any thickening on the shaft, may be subtle, so particularly feel where he tells you it bends.

Mature plaques may feel hard and "woody"

If you suspect penile suspensory ligament injury, palpate deeply at the base under the pubic arch. A defect of one or both of the ligaments may be discernible.

Check if he's circumcised or if the foreskin is tight (may affect later surgery).

Get him to come back with a photo of the erect penis. If he can't, consider a low dose (5 mcg) Alprostadil intra-cavernosal injection in a private clinic room.

Investigations

Particularly if there is any E.D., check Glucose, Cholesterol and Testosterone.

Ultrasound may not show an immature, non-calcified or minor plaque, but is better for more mature ones.

Doppler ultrasound with Alprostadil injection can check the vascular component of E.D.

Rarely, for complex plaque's, an MRI may be of use.

MRI can help look for suspensory ligament defects.

Chapter 15
Erectile Dysfunction

Nigel Borley

Overview

The definition of erectile dysfunction is persistent inability to achieve or maintain penile erection sufficient for satisfactory sexual performance [1]. However, erectile dysfunction may mean different things to different men and their partners. It is worth checking he doesn't mean premature or delayed ejaculation, difficulties with orgasm, dyspareunia or even a problematic foreskin.

A satisfactory erection requires sufficient blood flow, intact nerves, correct hormonal milieu and psychological arousal. The commonest, and most important cause of ED to rule out is any vascular problem. As the penile arteries are narrower than cardiac vessels, ED may herald vascular disease 5 years before symptoms of ischaemic heart disease develop [2].

Men may present with another symptom and only mention ED at the end of the consultation, but taboos are gradually being broken down.

Life stresses or relationship difficulties may play a part and it can be helpful and informative if the partner can be present for the consultation as well.

N. Borley, BM, MRCS, MS, FRCS (Urol)
Department of Urology, Chelsea and Westminster Hospital,
London, UK
e-mail: nigelborley@hotmail.com

B. Challacombe, S. Bott (eds.), *Diagnostic Techniques in Urology*,   131
DOI 10.1007/978-1-4471-2766-6_15,
© Springer-Verlag London 2014

The cause may be obvious, such as treatment for prostate cancer or pelvic surgery/trauma. Pro-active early treatment of ED following their cancer treatment is best [3].

Young men can have congenital venous insufficiency, they will have a life long history of short lived erections (due to venous leakage when the initial arterial surge subsides).

Occasionally men will have had significant trauma during intercourse, enough to disrupt the suspensory ligaments underneath the pubic arch. Men will still get erections but they will appear to be softer as the penis does not rise so far. They may also appear softer as the base is unstable. Men are often not forth coming about the initiating event, and it may only come to light when treatments inexplicably fail.

History

A detailed history is all important and can be rewarding if time is spent on taking it.

Duration and onset: gradual onset is suggestive of organic disease whereas sudden onset may be psychogenic (new partner, life events etc.).

Does he get a full early morning erection? Does the erection go down before penetration? Can he get a full erection for masturbation? All suggest a psychogenic cause.

General health: most importantly ask about a history of or risk factors for vascular disease (diabetes, hypertension, smoking, raised cholesterol, family history). Enquire about neurological conditions and symptoms including impaired mobility or dexterity (diabetes may again feature).

Libido: decreased libido and energy levels, weight gain may indicate a reduced testosterone as part of the metabolic syndrome in older men. In younger men it may represent hyperprolactinaemia.

Penis: does he have any penile deformity (possible Peyronie's disease) or a symptomatic (tight) foreskin? More rarely any history suggestive of fracture or priapism.

Drugs: many classes of drugs may adversely affect erections, including those treating underlying vascular disease. The use of nitrates is important for treatment options (PDE5i's are contra-indicated). Ask about alcohol and smoking. Recreational drugs may also be a factor.

LUTS: BPH is known as a risk factor for ED [4], prostate cancer if locally advanced may affect the cavernosal nerves.

Psychiatric: depression, anxiety, schizophrenia including their treatments, may be implicated.

Partner: their general health, particularly if they have undergone hysterectomy or mastectomy.

Examination

This will often be guided by clues in the history. It can also help build the rapport that helps the consultation.

General: obesity, muscle mass, hair distribution.

Cardiovascular: BP, pulses

Neurological: lower limb sensation, anal tone

Abdomen: hepatomegaly

Genitalia: penile shape and size, foreskin, testicular size, prostate

Investigation

The main point of investigation is to rule out treatable vascular and endocrine causes. The rest of the tests are reserved, if first line treatments of PDE5 inhibitors or PGE1 injections fail, and the cause is elusive.

For all: glucose and fasting cholesterol.

Testosterone (particularly if indicated from history). LH/FSH, prolactin, thyroid function, though the pick up may be low. If symptomatic of hypogonadism but total testosterone is normal, measure SHBG to check the free (available) fraction.

Doppler ultrasonography: an intra-cavernosal injection of PGE1 is necessary (though the patient may be too anxious for it to be effective in a radiology department). If the peak of the arterial wave is reduced (<20 cm/s) it may indicate arterial insufficiency. The flow in diastole should be zero, if it's >5 cm/s it may represent veno-occlusive dysfunction.

Nocturnal Penile Tumescence: men should get three or more erections during a night's sleep. If they don't it implies organic disease, if they do, it implies psychogenic ED. The test involves placing a ring at the base and tip of the penis to record circumference and rigidity. It's not diagnostic and can be affected by quality of sleep.

Advanced tests: may be helpful if there is previous pelvic injury or angioplasty is considered.

Cavernosometry and cavernosogram. Two canulae are inserted into the penis, one to infuse saline the other to measure pressure. An intracavernosal injection of PGE1 is given, an erection should be achieved if >100 ml/s is infused. If not, contrast is injected to identify any significant leaking veins.

Arteriography: the femoral artery is catheterized and the patency of the iliac vessels assessed. The internal pudendal artery may then be canulated to assess patency.

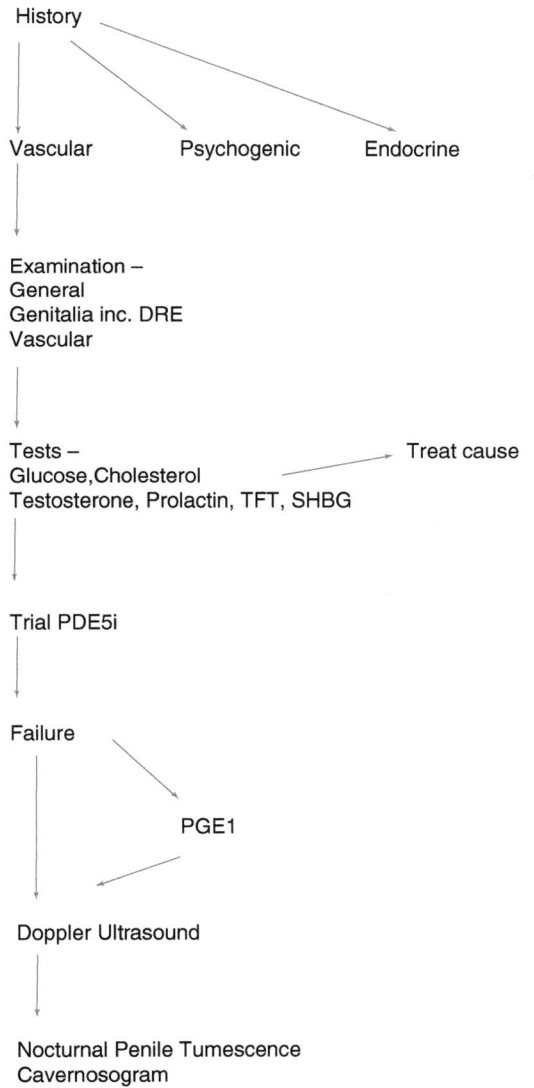

History

Vascular   Psychogenic   Endocrine

Examination –
General
Genitalia inc. DRE
Vascular

Tests –   Treat cause
Glucose,Cholesterol
Testosterone, Prolactin, TFT, SHBG

Trial PDE5i

Failure

PGE1

Doppler Ultrasound

Nocturnal Penile Tumescence
Cavernosogram
Arteriography

References

1. NIH Consensus Conference. NIH consensus development panel on impotence. JAMA. 1993;270:83–90.
2. Inman BA, et al. A population-based longitudinal study of erectile dysfunction and future coronary artery disease. Mayo Clin Proc. 2009;84:108.
3. Padma-Nathan H, McCullough AR, Levine LA, Lipshultz LI, Siegel R, Montorsi F, Giuliano F, Brock G. Randomized, double-blind, placebo-controlled study of postoperative nightly sildenafil citrate for the prevention of erectile dysfunction after bilateral nerve-sparing radical prostatectomy Sildenafil and ED after radical prostatectomy. Int J Impot Res. 2008;20:479–86. doi:10.1038/ijir.2008.33.
4. McVary KT. Erectile dysfunction and lower urinary tract symptoms secondary to BPH. Eur Urol. 2005;47(6):838–45.

Chapter 16
Male Infertility and OAT Syndrome

Nicholas Drinnan and Harry Naerger

Around one in six couples in the UK will seek medical therapy in order to combat infertility – defined by the World Health Organisation (WHO) as "the inability of a sexually active, non contracepting couple to achieve spontaneous pregnancy within 1 year," [1].

It is a complex problem where subfertility may only become apparent when both partners are affected. It is important, therefore, that both parties be considered simultaneously when referred for further investigation.

Oligospermia is defined as a deficiency of sperm cells within semen. The sperm count fluctuates even in healthy individuals, so consistently low readings on two separate occasions must be recorded before further investigation is begun. Historically concentrations below 20 million/ml were considered deficient, however more recently WHO have amended the reference limit to below 15 million/ml consistent with the 5th centile for fertile men.

Causes for the condition are numerous and are most clearly thought of anatomically – being Pre-testicular, Testicular and Post-testicular, as outlined in Table 16.1.

N. Drinnan • H. Naerger (✉)
Department of Urology, Frimley Park Hospital,
NHS Foundation Trust, Frimley, UK
e-mail: harry.naerger@fph-tr.nhs.uk

B. Challacombe, S. Bott (eds.), *Diagnostic Techniques in Urology*, 137
DOI 10.1007/978-1-4471-2766-6_16,
© Springer-Verlag London 2014

TABLE 16.1 Causes of oligospermia

Pre-testicular		Testicular		Post-testicular	
Inadequate hormonal or systemic support of testes		Inadequate production of semen by testes		Inadequate passage of semen through ejaculatory tract	
Genetic/congenital	Hypogonadism	Genetic/congenital	Y- microdeletion, klinefelters	Genetic/congenital	Abnormal Vas or ejaculatory duct
			Cryptorchidism		
			Testicular ysgenesis		
Infection	Sepsis	Infection	Mumps	Infection	Prostatitis
			Malaria		
Lifestyle	Obesity	Increased temperature	Varicocele	In all cases neoplasia and iatrogenic causes should be considered.	
	Smoking				
	Alcohol				
Systemic	Diabetes	Immunological	Autoimmune disease, Antisperm Ab		

In around 40 % of cases no causative factor is found. These patients are known as idiopathically infertile males. No abnormality is seen on physical examination and endocrine testing is normal. However, semen analysis reveals oligospermia often with slow moving (azenozo-) and abnormal (teratozo-) sperm. In combination the abnormalities define Oligo-Astheno-Teratozo-Spermia (OAT) syndrome.

Diagnosis

To categorize infertility, both female and male partners should be investigated simultaneously, as the female's status will of course be linked to the final outcome of any treatment given to the male.

A full medical history and comprehensive physical examination are considered standard for all referrals.

Standard assessment should also include Semen Analysis. If all results of this analysis are within range (see Table 16.2) then one sample is satisfactory to deem the male's fertility 'normal.' However, if the results fall outside of range then repeat analysis should be undertaken at least once before andrological investigations are arranged. In those men diagnosed with azoospermia or extreme OAT, it is important to rule out obstructive causes as discussed in Chap. 17.

Hints: Semen Analysis
Provide the patient with a sterile pot. Ask them to abstain from sexual intercourse or masturbation for 48 h. The sample must be produced by masturbation and must be deposited directly into the pot rather than being transferred from another container (e.g. condom). Ideally, the sample should be delivered to the laboratory within 1 h of production and should be kept warm (e.g. in a pocket) rather than left out in the cold (Table 16.2).

TABLE 16.2 Semen analysis reference limits

Parameter	Lower limit
Semen volume (mL)	1.5
Sperm concentration (106 per mL) (oligospermia)	15
Total motility (PR + NP, %) (asthenospermia)	40
Sperm morphology (normal forms, %) (teratospermia)	4
Total sperm number (106 per ejaculate)	39
Progressive motility (PR, %)	32
Vitality (live spermatozoa, %)	58

WHO Manual examination and processing of human semen, 5th edn, 2010

Causes and Investigation

Biochemical

Once diagnosed, all oligospermic men should undergo Hormonal Screening and Microbiological Assessment. Hormonal screening should include measurement of leutenising (LH) and follicle stimulating (FSH) hormones, in order to aid the diagnosis. As FSH and LH levels may fluctuate it is advisable to repeat the biochemical analysis if initial measurements are equivocal. For repeated equivocal levels further investigation may include testosterone levels (before 10 a.m.) and sex-hormone-binding (SHBH) hormone levels (inversely correlating to the amount of unbound, "free" testosterone) (Table 16.3).

Idiopathic hypo-gonadotrophic hypogandism is characterized by low levels of gondotrophin and sex steroid in the absence of anatomical or functional abnormalities of the hypothalamic-pituitary-gonadal axis. Genetic mutations can be found in 30 % of congenital cases and should be screened for prior to assisted reproduction. If unexplained hypo-gonadotrophic hypogonadism is present, Magnetic Resonance imaging (MRI) of the pituitary gland is indicated in order to rule out neoplasia.

TABLE 16.3 Causes of altered hormone levels associated with oligospermia

	Congenital	**Acquired**
Pre-testicular	Kallman syndrome	CNS tumour/ pituotary adenoma
Low LH/FSH	Prader Willi syndrome	Haemachromatosis
Hypothalamo-pituitary failure	Idiopathic	Iatrogenic
Hypo-gonadotrophic Hypogonadism		
Testicular	Klinefelter's syndrome	Orchitis
High LH/FSH	Cryptorchidism	Torsion
Testicular failure	Testicular dysgenesis	Testicular tumour
Hyper-gonadotrophic Hypoganodism	Y-microdeletion	Cytotoxic therapy

Ultrasonography

Ultrasonography is vitally important in the analysis of the sub-fertile male, with a number of testicular and post-testicular abnormalities identifiable – testicular tumours are found in 0.5 %, while varicoceles are seen in around 30 %. Post-testicular obstructive causes within the prostate (see Table 16.1) may be identified with transrectal ultrasound and is therefore indicated in those with associated low ejaculatory volume.

In many departments ultrasound is available in the outpatient setting and should therefore form part of the primary assessment of those referred with infertility.

Microbiology

Where post-testicular infection is suspected it is important that a thorough microbiological assessment be completed.

Urinary tract, prostatic and sexually transmitted infections may all result in decreased concentrations of sperm, through direct blockage or production of spermatotoxic free radicals. Neisseria gonorrhea and chlamydia as well as chronic infection of the prostate or seminal vesicles may be associated with post-testicular obstruction, white cells in the semen and a low ejaculatory volume. As such, urine diptick, microscopy & culture of urine and full sexual health screen are indicated.

Genetic Evaluation

Technological advances in medicine have meant that men with low sperm counts are now provided with a reasonable likelihood of paternity through techniques such as in-vitro fertilization and intra-cytoplasmic sperm injection. However, the sperm of such men shows an increased rate of DNA damage and genetic abnormalities. Indeed men with oligospermia demonstrate DNA damage within spermatozoa, reduced rates of natural conception and increased rates of early pregnancy loss. Given the complexity of spermatogenesis it is in fact likely that most idiopathic subfertility cases relate to genetic deficiencies and mutations. It is simply that, as yet, the causative changes have not been found.

Chromosomal abnormalities can be numerical or structural and the greater the number of abnormalities the greater the degree of spermatic deficiency. For those men with severe oligospermia (<5 million/ml) there is a significantly higher incidence of chromosomal abnormalities (4 %).

The most common abnormality of the sex chromosome is Klinefelter's Syndrome (trisomy 47 XXY) which affects around 15 % of men with azoospermia. As seen in Table 16.3 the syndrome is associated with hypergonado-trophic hypogonadism and is characterized by eunuchoid features with or without gynaecomastia, bilaterally shrunken testicles and decreased testosterone levels. Those couples with Kleinfelter's syndrome present show a significantly reduced number of normal embryos compared to controls and because

of the increased risk of genetic abnormalities pre-implanta-
tion analysis and amniocentesis should be carried out in specialist centres with subsequent counseling and specialist care.

The most common X-linked disorder relating to infertility
is Kallman syndrome, caused by a mutation in the KALIG-1
gene on Px22.3 and manifesting as anosmia, facial asymmetry,
cleft palate, colour blindness, deafness, maldescended testes
and renal abnormalities. The hypo-gonadotrophic hypogonadism can be relatively easily reversed with hormone therapy allowing normal contraception but, again, genetic
screening in a specialist centre is advised.

Y-linked disorders relate to microdeletions. Specifically,
microdeletions found in three regions of the Y chromosome
termed azoospermic factor (AZF) a, b and c. complete
removal of the AZFa region leads to Sertoli cell only syndrome, removal of AZFb to spermatogenic arrest and AZFc
to a number of difficulties from oligo- to azoospermia. After
conception any Y deletions are transmitted to any male off-
spring and genetic screening must therefore be carried out.
Because of the prevalence of these deletions screening
should also be undertaken in all patients with severe oligospermia (<5 million/ml) and azoospermia.

Low fertility associated with anatomically anomalies, such as
bilateral absence of the vas deferens may also denote underlying
genetic malformations with links between absence of the vas
and the cystic fibrosis transmembrane regulator gene. Cystic
fibrosis is a fatal autosomal recessive disorder but is the most
common genetic disease in Caucasians. More than three quar-
ters of men with congenitally absent vas when tested carry two
CFTR-gene mutations, located on chromosome 7. The gene
encodes a membrane protein which influences the formation of
the distal epididymis, vas, seminal vesicles and ejaculatory ducts.

Testicular Biopsy

Testicular biopsy is performed in the presence of a normal
testicular volume and normal hormone profile. It represents

TABLE 16.4 Classification of testicular insufficiency on biopsy

Classification	Pathological features
Hypo-spermato-genesis	Reduced number of reproducing spermatogonia
Maturational arrest	Arrest of any stage of spermatogenesis (sperma -togonia/-tocyte/-tide)
Germ cell absence	Sertoli cell only syndrome
Seminiferous tubule absence	Tubular sclerosis

the most invasive, and therefore, least frequent of the investigations discussed in this chapter and is generally reserved for those patients with severe OAT or complete azoospermia. Its aim is to distinguish between testicular insufficiency and post-testicular obstruction. In post-testicular obstruction, one would encounter normal biopsy results. Meanwhile testicular insufficiency may be classified as outlined in Table 16.4.

Spermatogenesis may be focal and therefore it is recommended that several samples be taken. Testicular sperm extraction (TESE) shows very good repeatability and is the technique of choice. Other approaches include microsurgery and percutaneous sampling. Microsurgical testicular sperm extraction may increase retrieval rates by opening the testis, excising tubules of larger diameter and using mincing or enzymatic digestion to facilitate sperm search. Percutaneous Epididymal Sperm Aspiration (PESA) results in lower retrieval rates and does not allow histological examination to detect for carcinoma in situ or malignancy.

Treatment

Counselling

In the first instance it is important to provide patients with constructive advice about measures to improve their lifestyle to increase the likelihood of their intrinsic fertility. A number

Table 16.5 Management of primary endocrinoloigcal pathologies

Abnormality	Management
High prolactin	Dopamine agonist
Hypo-gonadotrophic hypogonadism	[a]HCG + [b]HMG or FSH
Low testosterone	Tamoxifen or Clomophene

[a]Human-chorionic gonadotrophin
[b]Human menopausal gonadotrohpin

of activities involve exposure to increased scrotal temperatures (use of saunas, motorcycle riding), general states of exhaustion (marathon or strength sport training) or states of poor general health (smoking, alcohol excess). In turn each of these leads to impaired semen quality and resultant subfertility. Such is their effect that they may well demonstrate reversal and improved quality upon cessation of the activity.

Hormone Treatment

In cases of hormonal imbalance treatment occurs with varying degrees of success. Some primary endocrinological pathologies may be treated as outline below in Table 16.5. However there has been no proven improved pregnancy rate in men suffering from idiopathic OAT syndrome treated with steroids, androgens, prolactin inhibitors, anti-oestrogens or gonadotrophins.

For those where primary and secondary causes of hypogonadism have been excluded the therapy depends upon whether the goal is to achieve normal androgen levels or achieve fertility. Normal androgen levels and development of secondary sexual characteristics can be achieved relatively easily with androgen replacement therapy, with injectable, oral and transdermal testosterone preparations available. However these should be avoided in those wishing to conceive as they severely limit FSH / LH and decrease resultant fertility. The existing guidelines suggest that testosterone levels >12 nmol/L do not require substitution and <8 nmol/L would benefit from treatment. If levels do fall between these two values supplementation should be based upon the presence of symptoms.

The stimulation of sperm production requires treatment with human chorionic gonadotrophin (hCG) combined with recombinant FSH or human menopausal gonadotrophin. Once pregnancy has been established, patients can then return to testosterone substitution alone.

Surgical Treatment

As one would expect the majority of surgical treatments for subfertility are reserved for obstructive causes and azoospermia and are discussed elsewhere (Chap. 17)

The abnormal enlargement of the pampiniform plexus in the scrotum that characterizes a varicocele is a common abnormality with andrological implication of failure of testicular development and discomfort. It is diagnosed with clinical examination, confirmed by colour flow Doppler Ultrasound and can be classified as per the table in Table 16.6.

Varicoceles are present in around 12 % of adult men and around 25 % of men with abnormal semen analysis. The exact relationship with reduced fertility is unknown but it does appear to be associated, in some men, with progressive testicular damage from adolescence. It is thought that there may be varicocele-mediated oxidative stress leading to sperm DNA damage, a process which has been shown to reverse following varicocelectomy. However, controversy still exists as to whether repair results in more spontaneous pregnancies.

For those men found to be oligo- or asthenozo-spermic for 2 years or more with clinical varicocele, repair has been demonstrated to be of benefit. However, the simple presence of varicocele with normal semen analysis does not justify prophylactic treatment in order to maintain fertility, with no apparent benefit from treatment compared to observation. In light of this, semen analysis should be undertaken in all those with varociceles considering surgery.

Table 16.6 Classification of varicocele

Grade	Characteristics
Subclinical	Not palpable or visible
Grade I	Palpable only during valsalva
Grade II	Palpable at rest
Grade III	Visible at rest

Post-testicular partial obstruction of the genital tract caused by infection or cystic structures may be treated tranurethrally with resection or incision of the cyst or ejaculatory ducts and may lead to improved semen quality. Unfortunately the long term pregnancy rates following such surgery have varying success.

Further Post-Testicular issues may occur as a result of ejaculatory disorders, typically suspected when low ejaculatory volumes are encountered. Most commonly they are seen in neurological disease (spinal cord injury, multiple sclerosis) and iatrogenically (following prostatectomy sympathectomy or antidepressant therapy). Retrograde ejaculation aims is difficult to manage and often harvesting of spermatozoa from the post-ejaculatory urine is required. In anejaculation electroejaculation or vibrostimulation may be employed after referral to a specialist centre. Sadly, DNA fragmentation and poor motility frequently occur resulting in poor semen quality and in vitro-fertilization and ICSI are often required.

Prevention During Childhood
Cryptorchidism or undescended testes is the most common congenital abnormality of the male genitalia, found in around 5 % of newborn males. By the age of 3 months this rate spontaneously falls to 2 %. Its aetiology is multifactorial involving genetic and endocrinological disruption. Within the first year of life these maldescended

testes demonstrate degeneration of germ cells. During the second year the number of these cells declines. Because of this and in order to preserve spermatogenesis early treatment is recommended. While hormonal treatment with hCG was historically the management of choice, it has now been abolished due to increased levels of germ cell apoptosis and decreased spermatogenesis. Surgical treatment is now favored through orchidopexy within the first or second year of life. With early surgery comes improved testicular growth and improved spermatogenic activity.

By adulthood men with untreated bilateral cryptorchidism demonstrate rate of oligospermia of 31 %. While orchidopexy at this stage is unlikely to significantly improve paternity rates for those with cryptorchidism and azoospermia fixation may, on rare occasions, lead to appearance of spermatozoa within the ejaculate.

Reference

1. Cooper TG, Noonan E, von Eckardstein S, et al. World Health Organization reference values for human semen characteristics. Hum Reprod Update. 2010;16:231–45.

Chapter 17
Male Hypogonadism and Cryptorchidism

Michela Pisani, David J. Ralph, and Giulio Garaffa

Introduction

Male Hypogonadism and *Cryptorchidism* can be found in isolation or in the context of congenital or acquired conditions. This chapter focuses on the diagnosis of these conditions.

M. Pisani, MD
Department of Urology, Broomfield Hospital,
Court Road, Broomfield, Chelmsford, Essex CM1 7ET, UK

D.J. Ralph, FRCS (Urol)
Department of Urology, St Peter's Andrology,
The Institute of Urology, London, UK

G. Garaffa, MD, FRCS (Urol) (✉)
Department of Urology, Broomfield Hospital,
Court Road, Broomfield, Chelmsford, Essex, CM1 7ET, UK

St Peter's Andrology, The Institute of Urology, London, UK
e-mail: giuliogaraffa@gmail.com

B. Challacombe, S. Bott (eds.), *Diagnostic Techniques in Urology*,   149
DOI 10.1007/978-1-4471-2766-6_17,
© Springer-Verlag London 2014

Male Hypogonadism

Male Hypogonadism (from Greek *hypo-=under* and *gonad-ism=gonads*) is the complex of symptoms and signs related to androgen production deficiency. According to its aetiology it can be classified into acquired and congenital. *Acquired hypogonadism* is relatively common affecting 1:200 males with a progressive increase in prevalence with ageing (about 4 % of men aged 40–49 years and 20 % of men aged 70–79 years). Klinefelter's syndrome (XXY) is the most common cause of congenital hypogonadism and occurs in 1: 500–1,000 live births. According to its pathogenesis, hypogonadism can be then subdivided into primary, when it is due to testicular failure, secondary, when it is consequence of an insufficient secretion of gonadotrophin-releasing hormone (GnRH) and/ or gonadotrophin, and in androgen insensitivity syndrome, when is due to end-organ resistance.

A list of the more common conditions associated with androgen deficiency is given in Table 17.1.

Diagnosis

History and Physical examination

The clinical features of hypogonadism depend on time of onset, duration and degree of androgen deficiency. Physical examination includes the identification of associated extra-genital abnormalities. A lack of androgen action during fetal life leads to the most significant effects and a genetically male child can be born with female genitalia, ambiguous genitalia (neither male nor female), underdeveloped male genitalia with or without hypospadias, cryptorchidism. An onset later in life can lead to a delayed or incomplete pubertal development. The affected boys, usually aged between 11 and 20 years, typically present with small testes, deficient penile size, gynecomastia, deficient or diminished facial and body hair. Other characteristics include poor representation of skeletal muscles while arms and legs are elongated when compared to

TABLE 17.1 Conditions associated with androgen deficiency

Disorders associated with primary hypogonadism (testicular deficiency = hypergonadotropic hypogonadism)

Congenital

Testicular disgenesia, undescendend testis (or Cryptorchidism), anorchia, chromosomic abnormalities such as Klinefelter's syndrome, mixed gonadal dysgenesis, focal and complete germ cell aplasia such as Sertoli-only syndrome

Acquired

Abdominal and genital trauma, testicular torsion, surgery, post-orchitis (viral and bacterial), medications (sulfasalazine, antihypertensives, cytostatic drugs, cimetidine, antiandrogens, ketaconazole), medical and surgical castration for prostate cancer), toxins, irradiation, varicocele, chronic illness (respiratory, neurological, cardiac), idiopathic

Disorders associated with secondary hypogonadism (hypothalamic or pituitary origin = hypogonadotropic hypogonadism)

Congenital

Kallmann' Syndrome, CHARGE syndrome, Congenital adrenal hypoplasia (CAH), mutations of GnRH-receptor or GPR54 genes, Fertile eunuch syndrome, idiopathic hypogonadothropic hypogonadism (IHH), Prader- Willi's syndrome, Laurence-Moon-Biedl's syndrome,

Acquired

Pituitary tumors (adenoma, craniopharyngioma, germinoma), systemic disorders (haemochromatosis, sarcoidosis,), iatrogenic (radiotherapy, pituitary and hypothalamic surgery), functional (physical/psychological stress, weight changes, anabolic steroids, recreational drug abuse)

End-organ resistance to androgens

Luteinizing hormone (LH) receptor failure, Androgen resistance/absence state and enzyme defects such as CAIS (Complete Androgen Insensitivity syndrome or Morris's syndrome), PAIS (Incomplete androgen insensitivity or Reifenstein's syndrome), 5α Reductase deficiency

the size of the trunk due to a delay of epyphyseal closure (*eunuchoid habitus*). All these are classic features in boys who are diagnosed with Klinefelter's syndrome (47,XXY) and 47,XXY/46,XY mosaicism-variant (*primary hypogonadism* or *hypergonadotropic hypogonadism*). In Kallmann's syndrome (*idiopatic hypogonadotropic hypogonadism*), the lack of sense of smell (anosmia) is very common (>50 %) as well as the presence of other congenital malformations such as cleft lip and palate, senso-neural deafness, cerebellar ataxia and renal agenesis. Hypogonadism in adulthood or *late onset hypogonadism* (LOH), may lead to infertility (oligo- or azoospermia), lack of sexual drive and erectile dysfunction. General problems include weakness, muscle and bone loss, abdominal adiposity (central obesity), depressed mood and cognitive problems which if not early identified and left untreated, especially in congenital disorders, can lead to permanent problems. During physical examination, testes should be precisely described for position, volume (compared with standard Prader's orchidometer) and texture. Examination of the genitalia includes measurement of penile length, identification of possible presence of hypospadia and peno- scrotal transposition. The stage of puberty as well as the extent of virilization should be assessed and graded according to the Tanner criteria.

Laboratory Tests

Baseline serum testosterone levels and, after puberty, a semen analysis to assess the fertility potential represent the mainstay laboratory tests. Further tests may be required in presence of specific clinical findings. An early morning testosterone level >12 nmol/L (350 ng/dl) excludes a condition of hypogonadism while a normal semen analysis is generally indicative of good gonadal health. If serum testosterone levels are slightly inferior to normal at two controls (<12 nmol/L and >8 nmol/L) or the clinical finding do not match with the testosterone levels, free-testosterone (bioavailable testosterone) and sex hormone binding globulin (SHBG) should be checked. SHBG is inversely correlated with free-testosterone and can be influenced by systemic diseases. Conditions such as obesity, diabetes mellitus, nephrosic syndrome, hypothyroidism, androgens and glucocorticoids intake, Cushing's syndrome are known to decrease SHBG levels while hepatic cirrhosis, hyperthyroidism, oestrogen, androgen deficiency, anticonvulsants and HIV infection have the opposite effect. The levels of luteinizing hormone (LH) and follicle stimulating hormone (FSH) are used to distinguish between primary (hypergonadothropic hypogonadism) and secondary hypogonadism (hypogonadothropic hypogonadism). High FSH levels are highly indicative of precocious spermatogenesis arrest although up to 40 % of azoospermic men have normal FSH values. In pre-pubertal boys, gonadotropins are released in a more pulsatile fashion than in adults and therefore their levels are less reliable. Inhibin B, anti Mullerian hormone (AMH) and insulin-like factor 3 (INSL-3), glycoproteins secreted into the blood stream, are further markers of gonadal function. In particular, they tend to be low in primary testicular failure and normal in pituitary and hypothalamic dysfunctions. In Klinefelter's syndrome, FSH, LH, AMH, inhibin B, INSL-3 levels are usually normal before puberty and became progressively abnormal from mid-puberty. Kallmann's syndrome is characterized by low serum testosterone and gonadotropines which return to the normal range in response to GnRH administration. If a pituitary or hypothalamic condition is suspected, the serum levels of prolactin, cortisol, growth hormone (GH), thyroid stimulating hormone (TSH), insulin like growth factor 1 (IGF-1) and adrenocorticotropic hormone (ACTH) should be performed. Dynamic tests involving administration of human chorionic gonadotropin (hCG) or of luteinic hormone releasing hormone (LHRH) to stimulate the activity of the Leydig cells are of limited clinical value. In prepubertal boys with absent scrotal testes, a testosterone rise after administration of HCG indicates the presence of testes into the abdomen; in patients with no response to HCG stimulation, absence of the testes or Sertoli-only syndrome should be thought. If 5-reductase enzyme deficiency is suspected, dihydrotestosterone levels should be evaluated. When a congenital condition is suspected, chromosomal anomaly and/or a microdeletion in chromosome Y should be ruled out with a karyotype analysis and a testicular biopsy is recommended. In patients with confirmed hypogonadism, full blood count, lipid and sugar profiles as well as bone age should be assessed. This is because of the strong association between low testosterone levels, body composition and metabolic syndrome.

Imaging

Ultrasound scan should be performed to better assess the testicular volume and to identify abnormalities that may not been detected during physical exam (e.g. hydrocele, tumour). An MRI scan should be requested to demonstrate the presence of non- palpable testes or müllerian remnants such as a uterus. MRI scan in secondary hypogonadism can demonstrate the absence of the olfactory bulb in Kallmann's syndrome as well as the presence of pituitary tumours.

Cryptorchidism

Cryptorchidism (from the Greek "*kriptos*"="hidden" and "*orchis*"="testis") refers to the absence of the testis into the scrotum. Unilateral cryptorchidism is the most common disorder of sexual differentiation in the newborn, affecting 3 % of full-term males and about 30 % of premature neonates. The vast majority of cryptorchid testes will descend naturally in the scrotum within the first year of life, however its prevalence remains high in prematures, small size for gestational age newborns and siblings. In 10–30 % of cases it occurs bilaterally. A boy with unilateral cryptorchidism has a paternity chance of 90 %, the same of a boy with normal bilateral descended testes, while in bilateral undescended testes the paternity rate is less than 60 %.

Testis Descent

Once genes in both chromosome Y (SRY gene) and auto-somes have determined the sex of an individual, the gonads, which are situated beside the mesonephric kidneys, initiate to differentiate into testes and to produce male hormones. Anti-Mülleran hormone (AMH), secreted by the primitive Sertoli cells determines the regression of the Mülleran ducts while testosterone, produced by fetal Leydig cells, stimulates the Wolffian duct, precursor of the male genital tract. Testicular descent from the abdomen to the scrotum through the inguinal canal is completed between the 28th and 37th week of gestation. It is characterized by enlargement of the genito-inguinal ligament (or gubernaculums) and regression of the cranial suspensory ligament. The insulin-like hormone 3 (INL-3) produced by Leydig cells is thought to stimulate the caudal gubernaculum to grow, while AMH is responsible of the swelling reaction in the gubernaculum. A lack or a defective mechanism along this normal pathway can result in arrest of testicular descent. It has been postulated that environment and chemical factors such as synthetic/natural estrogens and pesticides act as endocrine disruptors during fetal life [ ] Furthermore, the major incidence in siblings and the association with congenital abnormalities, such as Prader-Willy's syndrome, Noonan's syndrome and cloacal and bladder exstrophy, suggests that there is also a genetic component.

Classification

Undescended testes can be found as *palpable* or *not-palpable. Palpable testes*, which account for up to 80 % of cases, can be *incompletely descended* within the inguinal canal or just outside the external inguinal ring or *ectopic*, when located in the superficial inguinal pouch between Scarpa's fascia and external oblique fascia (Denis Brown fascia) or along the perineal and femoral region. It has been postulated that ectopic testes have been misdirected outside the inguinal ring by an abnormal gubernaculum. *Non palpable testes* can be *intra-abdominal, inguinal* or *absent* (*vanishing testis* or *testicular agenesia*). *Retractile testes* are fully descended testes that are intermittently palpable outside the scrotum, usually along the inguinal area, as a result of an overactive cremasteric reflex. An *ascending testis* instead is a previously normal or retractile testis that has become high due to a short and tight spermatic cord preventing the testis from staying into the scrotum. It can be sometimes consequent to an inguinal hernia repair.

Diagnosis

History and Physical Examination

The best time to assess a patient with cryptorchidism is when he is less than 6 months of age, as the cremasteric reflex is weaker in the newborn. Physical examination should be extended to the whole body to note the possible presence of associated abnormalities. A normal shaped hemiscrotum suggests that the testis can be found below the external ring. Palpation should start above the scrotum by applying a firm pressure with one hand from the superior anterior iliac region towards the scrotum while the opposite hand is used to palpate the scrotum. Putting the child in a frog-legged position with the soles of his feet against each other allows an adequate relaxation of the cremaster muscle and therefore it represents the ideal position to examine the patient.

Laboratory Tests

An isolated unilateral cryptorchidism does not require laboratory tests. When unilateral and/or bilateral non-palpable testes are present in association with hypospadias, ambiguous genitalia and other anomalies, it is mandatory to exclude a life- threatening condition such as congenital adrenal hyperplasia (CAH). Blood electrolytes and glucose levels, hormonal profile as 17-OH progesterone (17OHP), plasma renin, D4 androstenedione, testosterone, 11-deoxy-cortisol and dehydroepiandrosterone (DHEA) should be evaluated as well as karyotype-analysis in these patients. In urine, the typical finding is an increase in the androgen metabolites (androstenedione, androsterone and etiochola-nolone, but it is unclear if this is reliable across all the age groups. A normal-looking phallus does not exclude this condition. Wolffian duct abnormalities have been reported in approximately 50 % of patients with undescended testes, including vasal and epididymal agenesis, segmental atresia and elongation. LH and FSH are commonly markedly high in absent testes. Typically, if a testis is present, testosterone levels raises after administration of hCG and LHRH, unless a Sertoli-only syndrome is present. AMH and Inhibin B dosage are complementary markers of gonadal function.

Imaging

Ultrasonography (US) is associated with low sensitivity and specificity to identify not- palpable testes. Computed tomography (CT) and gonadal vasography require exposure to ionizing radiations and therefore should not be offered. MRI is a very reliable test to demonstrate the presence or absence of non- palpable testes as well as Müllerian remnants such as a uterus, although it doesn't substitute surgical exploration.

Surgical Exploration

Laparoscopy is the gold standard diagnostic procedure in the identification of non palpable testes. It represents at the same time a diagnostic and therapeutic manoeuver, as it allows to place the testis into the scrotum. Therapy of cryptorchidism should be performed within the first year of life in order to prevent the irreversible deteriorations of testicular tissue, which is likely to occur after 12–18 months, with irreversible consequences on fertility and potential for cancer.

A multidisciplinary expert team including endocrinologists, surgeons, genetists, psychologists, neonatologists and nursing is mandatory to manage these issues.

Further Reading

1. Petak SM, Nankin HR, Spark RF, Swerdloff RS, Rodriguez-Rigau LJ; American Association of Clinical Endocrinologists. Medical Guidelines for Clinical Practice for the Evaluation and Treatment of Hypogonadism in Adult Male Patients: 2002 update. Endocr Pract. 2002; 8:440–56. Erratum in Endocr Pract. 2008;14(6):802–3.
2. Bojesen A, et al. Klinefelter syndrome in clinical practice. Nat Clin Pract Urol. 2007;4:192–204.
3. Bojesen A, Høst C, Gravholt CH. Klinefelter's syndrome, type 2 diabetes and the Metabolic syndrome: the impact of body composition. Mol Hum Reprod. 2010;16:396–401.
4. Bojesen A, et al. Morbidity in Klinefelter syndrome: a Danish register study based on hospital discharge diagnoses. J Clin Endocrinol Metabol. 2006;91:1254–60.
5. Sanders C, Simmonds M, Wallace AM, Watt A, Willis D. UK guidance on the initial evaluation of an infant or an adolescent with a suspected disorder of sex development. Clin Endocrinol (Oxf). 2011;75:12–26.
6. Chemke J, Carmichael R, Stewart JM, et al. Familial XY gonadal dysgenesis. J Med Genet. 1970;7:105–11.
7. Skakkebaek NE, Rajpert-De Meyts E, Main KM. Testicular dysgenesis syndrome: an increasingly common developmental disorder with environmental aspects. Hum Reprod. 2001;16(5):972–8.
8. De la Chapelle A. Nature and origin of males with XX sex chromosomes. Am J Hum Genet. 1972;24:71–105.
9. Demisch K, Nieckelsen T. Distribution of testosterone in plasma proteins during replacement therapy with testosterone enanhate in patient suffering from hypogonadism. Andrologia. 1983;15:536–41.
10. European Association of Urology Guidlines 2012 edition www.uroweb.org.

11. Faisal Ahmed S, Achermann JC, Arlt W, Balen A, Conway G, Edwards Z, Elford S, Hughes IA, Izatt L, Krone N, Miles H, O'Toole S, Perry L, Sanders C, Simmonds M, Michael Wallace A, Watt A, Willis D. UK guidance on the initial evaluation of an infant or an adolescent with a suspected disorder of sex development. Clin Endocrinol (Oxf). 2011. doi:10.1111/j.1365-2265.2011.04076.

12. Gearhart JP, Rink RC, Mouriquan PDE. Pediatric urology. 2nd ed. Philadelphia: Saunders/Elsevier; 2010.

13. Chavhan GB, Parra DA, Oudjhane K, Miller SF, Babyn PS, Pippi Salle FL. Imaging of ambiguous genitalia: classification and diagnostic approach. RadioGraphics. 2008;28:1891–904. doi:10.1148/rg.287085034.

14. Hadziselimovic F, Herzog B. Cryptochidism, its impact on male fertility. Horm Research. 2001;55(1):1–56.

15. Hameed A, Brothwood T, Bouloux P. Delivery of testosterone replacement therapy. Curr Opin Invest Drugs. 2003;4:1213–9. ChemPort.

16. Harman SM, Metter EJ, Tobin JD, Pearson J, Blackman MR. Longitudinal effects of aging on serum total and free testosterone levels in healthy men. Baltimore Longitudinal Study of Aging. J Clin Endocrinol Metab. 2001;86(2):724–31.

17. Heyns CF, Hutson JM. Historical review of theories on testicular descent. J Urol. 1995;153(3 Pt 1):754–67.

18. Krone N, Hughes BA, Lavery GG, et al. Gas chromatography/mass spectrometry (GC/MS) remains a pre-eminent discovery tool in clinical steroid investigations even in the era of fast liquid chromatography tandem mass spectrometry (LC/MS/MS). J Steroid Biochem Mol Biol. 2010;121:496–504.

19. Josso N, Nezelof C, Picon R, et al. Gonadoblastoma in gonadal dysgenesis: a report of two cases with 46,XY/45,XO mosaicism. J Pediatr. 1969;74:425–37.

20. Jost A. Recherches sur la differenciation sexuelle de l'embryon de lapin: III. Rôle des gonades fœtales dans la différenciation sexuelle somatique. Arch Anat Microsc Morph Exp. 1947;39: 271–315.

21. Kremer H, Kraaij R, Toledo SP, et al. Male pseudohermaphroditism due to a homozygous missense mutation of the luteinizing hormone receptor gene. Nat Genet. 1995;9:160–4.

22. Lanfranco F, et al. Klinefelter's syndrome. Lancet. 2004;364: 273–83.

23. Jongmans MCJ, van Ravenswaaij-Arts CMA, Pitteloud N, Ogata T, Sato N, der Grinten K, van der Donk K, Seminara S, Bergman

JEH, Brunner HG, Crowley Jr WF, Hoefsloot LH. *CHD7* mutations in patients initially diagnosed with Kallmann syndrome – the clinical overlap with CHARGE syndrome. Clin Genet. 2009;75(1):65–71.

24. Migeon CJ, Wisniewski AB. Human sex differentiation and its abnormalities. Best Pract Res Clin Obstet Gynaecol. 2003;17: 1–18.

25. Müller J, Ritzen EM, Ivarsson SA, et al. Management of males with 45, X/46, XY gonadal dysgenesis. Horm Res. 1999;52:11–4.

26. Nawras M, Jay S, Grace Y, Harry F, Ridwan S. Hypogonadism and Metabolic Syndrome: implications for testosterone therapy. J Urol. 2005;174:827–34. 0022-5347/05/1743-0827/0.

27. Nihoul-Fékété C, Lortat-Jacob S, Cachin O, Josso N. Preservation of gonadal function in true hermaphroditism. J Pediatr Surg. 1984;19:49–55.

28. Oppenheim DS, Greenspan SL, Zervas NT, Schoenfeld DA, Klibanski A. Elevated serum lipids in hypogonadal men with and without hyperprolactinemia. Ann Intern Med. 1989;111(4):288–92. Massachusetts General Hospital, Boston.

29. Radicioni AF, Ferlin A, Balercia G, Pasquali D, Vignozzi L, Maggi M, Foresta C, Lenzi A. Consensus statement on diagnosis and clinical management of Klinefelter syndrome. J Endocrinol Invest. 2010;33(11):839–50.

30. Rhoden EL, Morgentaler A. Risks of testosterone-replacement therapy and recommendations for monitoring. N Engl J Med. 2004;350(5):482–92.

31. Starceski PJ, Sieber WK, Lee PA. Fertility in true hermaphroditism. Adolesc Pediatr Gynecol. 1988;1:55–6.

32. Turner H, Wass J. Oxford handbook of endocrinology and diabetes. 2nd ed. Oxford/New York: Oxford University Press; 2009.

33. Yanagisawa S. Structural abnormalities of the Y chromosome and abnormal external genitalia. Hum Genet. 1980;53:183–8.

34. Yousem DM, Turner WJ, Li C, Snyder PJ, Doty RL. Kallmann syndrome: MR evaluation of olfactory system. AJNR Am J Neuroradiol. 1993;14(4):839–43.

Chapter 18
Renal Trauma

Kevin O'Connor and Declan G. Murphy

Introduction

Renal trauma is rare, accounting for only 0.3 % of trauma injuries [1]. It is the third most commonly injured abdominal organ after the spleen and liver, accounting for 10 % of patients who sustain abdominal trauma [2]. The mechanism of renal injury is classified as either blunt or penetrating with the vast majority (81 %) resulting from blunt trauma [1]. A relatively higher incidence of penetrating renal injuries are encountered in an urban setting. Coexisting injuries are identified in 14–34 % of blunt trauma and in 50–80 % of penetrating renal trauma cases [3]. Renal trauma can be acutely life threatening necessitating immediate surgical exploration,

K. O'Connor
Department of Urology, Royal Melbourne Hospital,
Melbourne, VIC Australia

D.G. Murphy (✉)
Division of Cancer Surgery, Peter MacCallum Cancer Centre,
University of Melbourne, East Melbourne,
VIC 3002, Australia
e-mail: declan.murphy@petermac.org

B. Challacombe, S. Bott (eds.), *Diagnostic Techniques in Urology*,   161
DOI 10.1007/978-1-4471-2766-6_18,
© Springer-Verlag London 2014

but the majority of renal injuries are not severe and can be managed conservatively. The management of renal injuries has changed over time with a tolerance for a non-operative approach, even in the most seriously injured kidneys.

Initial Assessment

The initial assessment of the patient should be in accordance with the Advanced Trauma Life Support (ATLS) proto- cols, focusing on the rapid identification and stabilization of life-threatening injuries. Direct history is obtained from conscious patients, paying particular attention to flank or abdominal pain in association with haematuria. Witnesses and emergency personnel can provide valuable information regarding the unconscious or seriously injured patients. The mechanism of injury provides the framework for the clinical assessment. Possible indicators of major renal injury include a rapid deceleration event (fall, high-speed motor vehicle accidents) and a direct blow to the flank. In penetrating inju- ries, important information includes the size of the weapon in stabbings and the type and caliber of the weapon used in gun- shot wounds since high-velocity projectiles have the potential for more extensive damage especially at close range. Past renal surgery, and known pre-existing renal abnormalities such as pelvic-ureteric junction (PUJ) obstruction, large cysts and stones should be recorded.

Haemodynamic stability is the primary criterion for the management of all renal injuries. Haemodynamic instability is defined as a systolic blood pressure of less than 90 mmHg found at any time during an adult patient's evaluation. A thorough examination of the thorax, abdomen, flanks and back for penetrating wounds should be performed. Key find- ings on physical examination that could indicate possible renal injury include haematuria, flank abrasions and ecchy- mosis, seat belt marks, fractured ribs, abdominal tenderness, distension or mass.

Children are more susceptible to renal injuries as their kidneys lie lower in the abdomen, with less protection from the lower ribs. They also have less cushioning due to the paucity of perirenal fat. A high index of suspicion for renal trauma is required in the paediatric population as unlike adults, significant injury can be present despite a stable blood pressure [4]. Another important difference from adults is that children with microscopic haematuria and stable vital signs may have sustained significant renal injury [5]. Often trivial abdominal trauma leading to haematuria can be the first presentation of a renal condition such as a PUJ obstruction [6].

Laboratory Tests

Urinalysis, haematocrit and baseline creatinine are the most important tests for evaluating renal trauma [7]. Falling serial haematocrit measurements help indicate ongoing blood loss. Microscopic haematuria in the trauma setting may be defined as greater than five red blood cells per high power field (RBC/HPF), while gross haematuria is demonstrated by urine in which blood is readily visible. Although haematuria is a hallmark sign for renal injury, it is neither sensitive nor specific enough for differentiating minor and major injuries. Initial creatinine measurement could highlight patients who had impaired renal function prior to injury.

Radiographic Assessment

Contrast enhanced computerised tomography (CT) is the imaging modality of choice once the patient has been stabilised. CT is more sensitive and specific than intravenous urogram (IVU), ultrasonography or angiography. It confirms the presence of renal and associated intra-abdominal injuries and defines their extent. In order to complete the proper evaluation and staging of renal injuries after imaging in the arterial and venous phase, later imaging in the nephrogram phase (>80 s) is needed to detect renal parenchymal and venous injury, while delayed images (2–10 min) are required to detect ureteral and PUJ injuries. Ultrasonography may be used at the beside of a trauma patient to look for free fluid as part of Focused Assessment by Sonography in Trauma (FAST). It provides a quick, non invasive, low cost means of detecting free fluid in the peritoneal cavity without radiation exposure. Ultrasound is however highly operator dependent and often blood in the peritoneal cavity can lead to difficulty in obtaining good acoustic windows. Even in well trained hands the true depth and extent of the renal injury cannot be definitely assessed.

All penetrating renal and hemodynamically unstable blunt renal trauma patients who require immediate surgical exploration should undergo one-shot, high-dose IVU prior to any renal exploration. In the situation of an unstable patient who emergently undergoes a laparotomy and a renal injury is suspected they should undergo an on table one shot IVU. A one-shot trauma IVU consists of a bolus intravenous injection of 2 mL/kg of radiographic contrast, followed by a single abdominal radiograph 10 min later. It provides important information for decision-making in the critical time of urgent laparotomy concerning the injured kidney, as well as determining the presence of a normal functioning kidney on the contralateral side.

Classification of Renal Trauma

Classifying renal injuries helps to standardise different groups of patients, select appropriate therapy and predict results. The American Association for the Surgery of Trauma (AAST) has developed a renal-injury grading system which is most commonly used [8]. Renal injuries are classified as grade 1–5 (Table 18.1). Abdominal CT or direct renal exploration is used to classify injuries (Fig. 18.1).

Management

Overall 95 % of blunt and 50 % of penetrating injuries can be managed non-operatively [5]. Following grade 1–4 blunt renal trauma, stable patients should be managed

TABLE 18.1 The American Association for the Surgery of Trauma Organ Injury Severity Scale

Grade[a]	Type	Description
I	Contusion	Microscopic or gross hematuria, urologic studies normal
	Hematoma	Subcapsular, nonexpanding without parenchymal laceration
II	Hematoma	Nonexpanding perirenal hematoma confined to renal retroperitoneum
	Laceration	<1 -cm parenchymal depth of renal cortex without urinary extravasation
III	Laceration	>1 -cm parenchymal depth of renal cortex without collecting system rupture or urinary extravasation
IV	Laceration	Parenchymal laceration extending through renal cortex, medulla, and collecting system
	Vascular	Main renal artery or vein injury with contained hemorrhage
V	Laceration	Completely shattered kidney
	Vascular	Avulsion of renal hilum, devascularizing the kidney

[a]Advance one grade for bilateral injuries up to grade III

conservatively with bedrest, hydration, prophylactic antibiotics and continuous monitoring of vital signs until haematuria resolves. Indications for surgical intervention include haemodynamic instability; expanding or pulsatile peri-renal haematoma identified at time of laparotomy; grade 5 injury and incidental finding of pre-existing renal pathology requiring surgical therapy [7].

The goal of renal exploration following renal trauma is control of haemorrhage and renal salvage. Most experienced authors advocate the transperitoneal approach for surgery as opposed to accessing the renal vessels through the

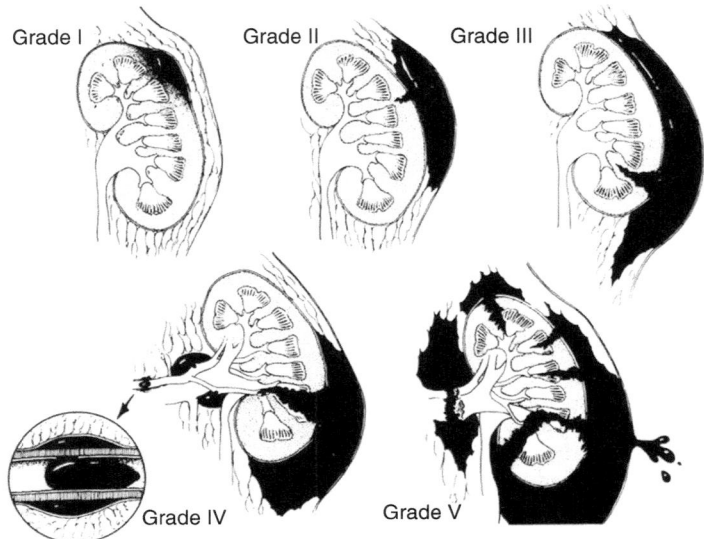

FIGURE 18.1 Grading of renal trauma according to American Association for the Surgery of Trauma Organ Injury Severity Scale

extraperitoneal space via a flank incision [2, 9]. Access to the renal vascular pedicle through the transperitoneal approach is obtained through the posterior parietal peritoneum, which is incised over the aorta, just medial to the inferior mesenteric vein. Temporary vascular occlusion before opening Gerota's fascia is a safe and effective method during exploration and renal reconstruction. It tends to lower blood loss and the nephrectomy rate.

Angiography is both diagnostic and therapeutic but is always performed after a CT. Angiography with selective renal embolisation for haemorrhage control is a reasonable alternative to laparotomy provided that no other indication for immediate surgery exists. Selective renal embolization is of particular benefit in iatrogenic penetrating renal injuries. A significant bleed post percutaneous nephrolithotomy (PCNL) requiring transfusion or selective renal embolization can be encountered in up to 10 and 1 % of patients undergoing this procedure respectively [10]. Non-operative management can lead to delayed complications especially in the higher-grade injuries (Grade 3–5). Repeat imaging 2–4 days after trauma minimises the risk of missed complications. Repeat imaging is always recommended in cases of fever, flank pain, or falling haematocrit. Perinephric fluid collections or urinomas are ameniable to percutaneous drainage. Persistent urinary extravasation often responds to ureteric stent insertion antegradely or retrogradely.

Follow Up

Within 3 months of major renal injury, patients' follow-up should involve: physical examination; urinalysis; individualised radiological investigation; serial blood pressure measurement and estimated GFR. Delayed complications include bleeding, hydronephrosis, calculus formation, chronic pyelonephritis, hypertension, arteriovenous fistula, hydronephrosis, and pseudoaneurysms. Arterial hypertension is an uncommon complication of renal trauma, although reports on its incidence vary from 1 to 40 %. Despite the relative scarcity of this complication, its potential negative impact on life expectancy and morbidity makes it a serious complication [11]. Hypertension may occur acutely as a result of external compression from peri-renal haematoma (Page kidney), or chronically because of compressive scar formation (Goldblatt kidney). Hypertension is caused by excess renin excretion which occurs following renal ischaemia. Arteriovenous fistulae usually present with delayed onset of significant haematuria, most often after penetrating trauma. Percutaneous embolisation is often effective for symptomatic arteriovenous fistulae, but larger ones may require surgery. The development of pseudoaneurysm is a rare complication following blunt renal trauma. In numerous case reports, transcatheter embolisation appears to be a reliable minimally invasive solution.

References

1. Hotaling JM, Wang J, Sorensen MD, et al. A national study of trauma level designation and renal trauma outcomes. J Urol. 2012;187(2):536–41.
2. McAninch JW. Genitourinary trauma. World J Urol. 1999; 17(2):65.
3. Santucci RA, Wessells H, Bartsch G, et al. Evaluation and management of renal injuries: consensus statement of the renal trauma subcommittee. BJU Int. 2004;93(7):937–54.
4. Quinlan DM, Gearhart JP. Blunt renal trauma in childhood. Features indicating severe injury. Br J Urol. 1990;66(5):526–31.
5. Angus LD, Tachmes L, Kahn S, Gulmi F, Gintautas J, Shaftan GW. Surgical management of pediatric renal trauma: an urban experience. Am Surg. 1993;59(6):388–94.
6. Sebastia MC, Rodriguez-Dobao M, Quiroga S, Pallisa E, Martinez-Rodriquez M, Alvarez-Castells A. Renal trauma in occult ureteropelvic junction obstruction: CT findings. Eur Radiol. 1999;9:611–5.
7. http://www.uroweb.org/gls/pdf/22_Urological_Trauma_LR%20II.pd
8. Moore EE, Shackford SR, Pachter HL, et al. Organ injury scaling: spleen, liver, and kidney. J Trauma. 1989;29:1664.
9. Nash PA, Bruce JE, et al. Nephrectomy for traumatic renal injuries. J Urol. 1995;153:609.
10. Martin X, Murat FJ, Feitosa LC, et al. Severe bleeding after nephrolithotomy: results of hyperselective embolization. Eur Urol. 2000;37:136–9.
11. Pereira Jr GA, Muglia VF, Dos Santos AC, Niyake CH, et al. Late evaluation of the relationship between morphological and functional renal changes and hypertension after non-operative treatment of high-grade renal injuries. World J Emerg Surg. 2012;7(1):26.

Chapter 19
Ureteric Injuries

Dan Wood

Introduction

The ureters are the tubular connection between the renal pelvis and the bladder. The have a serosal covering, a smooth muscle layer and a mucosal lining. They follow a retroperitoneal course crossing the sacroiliac joint, the iliac vessels and round the pelvic sidewall into the bladder. The anterior relations are the pancreas and duodenal-jejunal junction on the left. On the right the duodenum lies anteriorly and the IVC just medially. The vascular supply to the mid and hind gut cross the right and left ureter respectively, both pass in front of the iliac vessels but are crossed anteriorly by the gonadal vessels.

In the male pelvis they run behind the medial umbilical ligament and under the vas deferens. In females they lie behind the ovary but medial to the ovarian vessels, lateral to the infundibulopelvic ligament. They run behind the broad ligament and lateral to the uterus (1–2 cm lateral to the cervix) and behind the uterine vessels.

D. Wood, PhD, FRCS (Urol)
Department of Adolescent and Reconstructive Urology,
University College London Hospitals, London, UK
e-mail: danwood1@btinternet.com

B. Challacombe, S. Bott (eds.), *Diagnostic Techniques in Urology*,   169
DOI 10.1007/978-1-4471-2766-6_19,
© Springer-Verlag London 2014

Classification

- **Iatrogenic**
  - Obstructive
  - Perforation/Transection

- **Traumatic**
  - Blunt (less than 1 % of cases)
  - Penetrating (less than 4 % of cases)

- **Other**
  - Chemical
  - Inflammatory

Presentation

The most common ureteric injuries are iatrogenic and since urologists operate on the ureters the most it is not surprising that it is they that cause the most damage.

There are three types of endoscopic ureteric injury:

- Delayed stricture
- Perforating
- Avulsion

The rate of ureteric injury following ureteroscopy has fallen dramatically and is now quoted at around 1–5 % [1]. With the advent of better cameras and smaller 'ureteroscopes the injury rate comes down. The use of guidewires either through or alongside scopes further improves safety. A significant factor is the recognition of injuries, the need to place a stent and abandon any further attempt to continue – understanding this has reduced sequelae. As with many other procedures risk factors for endoscopic injury include inexperience of the surgeon, previous radiotherapy and longer procedure time [2, 3].

TABLE 19.1 Classification of Ureteric Injuries (adapted from the current management of renal injuries. American Association of Surgery, 2008 [1])

Grade	Description
I	Contusion
II	Transection <50 %
III	Transection >50 %
IV	Complete Transection <2 cm devascularisation
V	Avulsion >2 cm devascularisation

Traumatic Injuries

These are rare but when identified are often associated with other injuries that may result in mortality in up to 1/3 of cases [4].

A high index of suspicion is important in recognizing such injuries and other injuries may be significant factor in directing the mode and timing of treatment.

Such injuries to the ureter have been classified as accepted by the American Association for Surgery (Table 19.1).

Other Surgical Injuries

Type of surgery	% of ureteric injuries
Hysterectomy	54
Colorectal	14
Other pelvic surgery	8
Vascular	6

Management

Recognition/Diagnosis

Ideally a surgical injury is recognized and diagnosed immediately and depending on the type of injury different strategies can be employed.

Open Surgical Injury

In many ways these are the most straightforward scenarios if recognition is immediate. Some surgeons will request routine pre-operative ureteric stenting if they anticipate ureteric involvement in a lesion. There is no evidence that this reduces the rate of injury but it may increase the rate of recognition when an injury occurs. Of course this observation may be biased by the fact that those who request stenting are more aware of the risk of ureteric injury and therefore more likely to recognize such an injury in the first place.

A clean surgical transection of the ureter can be repaired in situ – a judgement must be made about the ureteric ends and surrounding tissues but if this appears healthy then debridement, spatulation and suture using 4/0 monocryl over a 6 french stent produces a good result. The time for stent removal is often a matter of preference but 4 weeks seems reasonable. More widespread tissue trauma involving the ureter may involve resection or abandonment of damaged tissue and in the lower to middle third this may be treated by ureteric reimplantation into the bladder with contralateral division of the superior vesical pedicle and an ipsilateral psoas hitch with a Boari flap if necessary. Some surgeons report Boari flaps that have been used to bridge a ureteric defect right up to the renal pelvis. This may be possible with a good volume bladder that mobilises well but the uretero-vesical anastomosis must be tension free otherwise the risk is a further anastomotic stricture. If this is not possible two options exist – either ileal interposition (a segment of ileum is taken on its mesentery and anastomosed to proximal healthy ureter and bladder) or transuretero-ureterostomy (TUU) (where the proximal segment of damaged ureter is passed behind the bowel mesentery and anastomosed (end-to-side) with the intact contralateral ureter). Both of these can be difficult and in the hands of a surgeon not familiar with reconstructive techniques may be unreasonable to take on. If in doubt it is safer to drain the kidney – either with a nephrostomy (standard treatment and definitely the first preference) or if this is not available an in situ, intubated end ureterostomy (a feeding or nasogastric tube tied into the ureter and brought out through the skin) will allow the patient to be woken up and transferred to a unit with the necessary expertise.

Once surgical reconstruction has been achieved and a stent removed the kidney will need to be monitored with a MAG renogram to ensure unobstructed drainage and an ultrasound to ensure a normal appearance of the kidney.

Endoscopic, Obstructing Injuries and Delayed Recognition

Whilst the mechanism for each of the above may be very different the principles of diagnosis and treatment are often very similar. A post-operative patient who develops loin pain needs evaluation with baseline bloods and an ultrasound. A hydronephrosis seen on ultrasound will necessitate a cystoscopy and bilateral retrograde study (very embarrassing to diagnose and treat one side and miss an occult injury on the other side). If a stent can be inserted at this time this may be enough to buy time or even treat the situation (about 50 % will settle following stent placement). The value of further imaging prior to this is questionable and will vary with the scenario but a contrast CT is not unreasonable if additional information is needed. If a stent cannot be placed a nephrostomy will be required and in expert uro-radiological hands an antegrade stent may be passable.

Similar principles can be applied to the post-operative urine leak. Following placement of a urethral catheter, a CT urogram will give more information than an ultrasound. Bilateral retrograde studies and potential stenting may still be possible and helpful – careful cystoscopy will help to exclude a bladder injury.

In all scenarios where a return to theatre for cystoscopy and retrogrades is planned it is worth discussing the merits of immediate open repair. If a defect cannot be stented and the time frame is reasonable (ie less that 2 weeks post procedure) then this may be the most sensible option. Unless the injury is a clean cut a psoas hitch, Boari flap, TUU or ileal interposition will be needed. Beyond 2 weeks after an open procedure the tissues will be very fragile and difficult to work with, making surgical repair risky. Once this time frame has elapsed a delayed repair is the better option – many surgeons would now wait up to 6 months before attempting reconstruction.

Occasionally, a short stricture as a result of a suture may be treated endoscopically using a laser – there is little data about long-term outcomes for this but it is certainly a reasonable option. Memocath stent placement is often possible but in stone formers or young patients whilst placement may be possible, the risk of encrustation or the subsequent change of management to a reconstructive option will certainly not be made easier. It is possible that encrustation and replacement or simply initial placement will lengthen a stricture and make subsequent reconstruction more complex as a result – patients need to be warned of this.

A ureteric avulsion will need an open reconstruction – the tissue will be ischaemic, therefore either a psoas hitch, Boari flap, TUU or ileal interposition will be needed depending on the point of detachment. There is no shame in placing a nephrostomy, waking the patient up and waiting for the correct person to be present to undertake such a repair. This allows the surgeons involved to explain what has and what will happen to the patient and to undertake the repair in a controlled environment with all the correct team and necessary equipment.

Summary

In short, awareness of the potential to injure a ureter and recognition of the injury are key. Diagnosis is important and if an injury one side is obvious don't forget to examine the other side to rule out a further occult injury. If necessary a nephrostomy will create a temporary (and usually not complete) urinary diversion and may allow for antegrade stenting. Either antegrade or retrograde stenting may be sufficient treatment. Beyond this in any other situation except a clean cut or single suture ligation open reconstruction, with options discussed, remains the gold standard. We may see the development of minimally invasive techniques with time but their widespread role remains to be established.

References

1. Voelzke BB, McAninch JW. The current management of renal injuries. Am Surg. 2008;74:667–78.
2. Brandes S, Coburn M, Armenakas NA, McAninch JW. Diagnosis and management of ureteric injury: an evidence based analysis. BJU Int. 2004;94:277–89.
3. Sommertom D, et al. European guidelines on urological trauma. 2013. p 32–5.
4. McAninch JW, Santucci RA. In: Campbell-Walsh urology. Wein AJ, Kavoussi LR, Novick AC, et al. (eds.). Renal and ureteral trauma. 9th ed. Philadelphia: Saunders Elsevier; 2007. p 1274–93.

Chapter 20
Penoscrotal Trauma

Andrew Chetwood and Ben Eddy

Introduction

Penoscrotal trauma can be isolated or associated with major abdominopelvic injury. Management should be prompt and under specialist care to ensure a good functional and cosmetic outcome. Injuries can be classified as blunt, penetrating or gunshot. This chapter aims to describe the common presentations of trauma to the external male genitalia with a focus on the diagnostic and management pathways.

If the scrotal trauma is associated with major abdomino-pelvic trauma management should part of ATLS International Trauma guidelines with penoscotal assessment as part of the secondary survey

Penile Trauma

Diagnosis can usually be made quickly in all cases from history and examination

A. Chetwood, BMedSci (Hons), MBChB (Hons), MRCS (✉)
Department of Urology, Frimley Park Hospital, Frimley, UK
e-mail: andrewchetwood@doctors.org.uk

B. Eddy, FRCS (Urol)
Department of Urology, Kent and Canterbury Hospital, Canterbury, UK

B. Challacombe, S. Bott (eds.), *Diagnostic Techniques in Urology*,   177
DOI 10.1007/978-1-4471-2766-6_20,
© Springer-Verlag London 2014

Penile Fracture (Rupture)

Penile fracture comprises rupture of the tunica albuginea of the penis leading to the extravasation of blood from the highly vascular corpora cavernosa. It only occurs in the erect penis.

The history usually comprises pain, a 'popping sound' and rapid detumescence usually occurring during intercourse with either compression of the penis against the partner's pubic bone on slipping out of the vagina, or during excessive angulation during intercourse. There have been reported cases of fracture during vigorous masturbation and in young men who have attempted to 'click' their penis to terminate their erection. The patient will complain of a sudden sharp pain, immediate swelling and loss of erection.

Examination reveals characteristic bruising confined to the penis ('the aubergine sign') but if Buck's fascia is compromised it may extend much further into the scrotum, perineum and anterior abdominal wall. There may be gross deformity and angulation of the penis. Blood at the meatus, at the start of the stream or urinary retention suggests concomitant urethral injury. There should be a high index of suspicion for this injury and ascending urethrogram or flexible urethroscopy should be used to rule it out, this has been reported in up to 20 % of cases [1]. Differential diagnosis of penile fracture includes ruptured dorsal penile veins or rupture of the penile suspensory ligament. Urethral injuries require repair over a catheter at surgery with a tension free, end-to-end urethral anastomosis.

Usually the diagnosis is clear, but imaging, either ultrasound or MRI can be used if the diagnosis is uncertain or to localise the tunica defect and origin of the haematoma, although a negative scan does not rule out the injury and injury should still be suspected on presentation. Surgical repair via a de-gloving circumferential or peno-scrotal incision is the standard technique and after evacuation of the haematoma the tear in the tunica can be closed using non-absorbable sutures. A longitudinal incision over defect can also be used although must allow adequate urethral exposure. In severe cases urethra and both cavernosal bodies may be involved. Delayed repair (after 24–36 h) or conservative management is not advocated as it can lead to higher rates of penile deformity, plaque formation or erectile dysfunction.

Amputation

Penile amputation is very rare. Diagnosis is usually obvious from history and examination. Initial management requires resuscitation and prompt haemostasis from the highly vascular corpora cavernosa. Patients may present with shock secondary to significant blood loss and require transfusion and urgent surgery. The aetiology consists primarily of assault but urologists should be alert to self-mutilation and the need for psychiatric input. The severed penis should be kept in a 'non-contact' manner in ice and microsurgical reconstruction should be performed as soon as possible. Warm ischaemia times of greater than 18 h are associated with poor results [2]. Supra-pubic urinary diversion may be required depending on the extent of the injury.

Reconstruction comprises initial closure of urethra over a catheter (two layer) with minimal dissection along neurovascular bundles. Re-approximation of cavernosal artery with 11-0 prolene (if possible) is followed by closure of tunica albuginea. The dorsal artery, vein and epineurium should be repaired with 11-0/9-0/10-0 nylon/prolene respectively [3]. If initial reconstruction is not sufficient then specialist involvement may be required with an aim to avoid perineal urethrostomy.

Bites

These are caused by either animals (commonly dogs) or humans and can involve paediatric patients. The main concern is infection which can be complicated by un-familiar pathogens. Initial treatment comprises broad spectrum antibiotics, protection against tetanus and rabies in conjunction with copious irrigation and debridement if required. Smaller wounds can be managed conservatively but larger defects may require delayed reconstruction once local infection has resolved. Once again the possibility of co-existing urethral injury should be considered and this can be associated with significant sequelae if left unrecognised including urethral strictures and urethra-cutaneous fistulae.

Penetrating Trauma

This is usually secondary to gun-shot or stab wounds during an assault. Patients often have multiple injuries and require initial assessment as per ATLS protocol.

Diagnosis is made from history and examination. Imaging is rarely helpful, although urethrogram or flexible urethroscopy can be used to rule out associated urethral injury. Surgical exploration of the penis is almost always required and, in contrast to bite wounds, following adequate wound toilet primary closure may be acceptable. Urinary diversion via a supra-pubic catheter can be required if there are concerns with wound contamination or urethral injuries.

De-gloving Injuries

This usually follows an industrial accident and skin loss can be extensive. Management comprises evaluation of co-existing injuries and irrigation and debridement of the wound. Minor injuries can be repaired primarily, with more extensive injuries split-thickness skin grafts can be used to cover the defect. Larger defects should be managed in a multimodality setting with plastic surgical input.

Burns either electrical or chemical are rare although can be extensive, diagnosis is usually clear. Electrical burns should be managed with fluid resuscitation, wound debridement and primary or secondary repair depending on the size of defect. Chemical burns should first be managed with extensive wound toilet. Urinary diversion with a suprapubic catheter should also be considered.

Strangulation

Patient will present with a constricting object at the base of the penis. Most commonly this consists of a ring placed during sexual activities to enforce erection and their removal complicated by distal penile oedema. It can also be seen with consticting rings used with vacuum devices. Removal may require lubrication and metal cutters with or without local anaesthesia. Care must be taken not to damage underlying penile skin and the urethra as it lies just under the skin on the ventral aspect of the shaft. Debridement of necrotic skin and subsequent split skin grafting maybe required in extreme cases.

Scrotal

Blunt Trauma

Preservation of spermatogensis and endocrine function form the basis of treating scrotal injuries. The exposed nature of the scrotum makes it vulnerable to injury but the mobility and elasticity of scrotal skin serves to protect from significant injuries.

Testicular Trauma

In the UK the most common causes are road traffic accidents and sports injuries, a history of "crushing" against the pubic rami suggests rupture. Patients present with scrotal pain and may have associated nausea and vomiting. Clinical examination may reveal bruising, a tender testis or skin damage. Ultrasound forms the mainstay of imaging and can examine the echotexture of the testes, vascularity and integrity of the tunica albuginea. A 5 mHz probe gives the best penetration. Ultrasound is operator dependent and it's accuracy in diagnosing testicular rupture has been quoted as being specificity 75 %, sensitivity 64 %, positive predictive value 78 % and negative predictive value 60 % [4]. Ultimately, if there is any doubt over the integrity of a testes or the ultrasound suggests rupture then urgent exploration is required. Conservative management of testicular rupture is not recommended.

The majority of blunt scrotal trauma comprises post-traumatic haematomas, hydroceles and contusion and should be managed conservatively with elevation, ice and analgesia. If testicular rupture is suspected then a midline raphe incision should be used to access the testicle. Any haematoma should be evacuated and extruding/necrotic testicular tissue requires debridement. Following wound cleaning the tunica albuginea can be repaired using an absorbable 4/0 suture. Drain placement should also be considered. Surgical exploration should be performed within 3 days with reported rates of testicular salvage beyond this falling from 90 % to below 45 % [5]. It should be noted that both testicular torsion and dislocation (subcutaneous or internal) can occur following scrotal trauma with both requiring surgical repair.

Penetrating Trauma

As for penetrating penile trauma there is an association with other potentially life-threatening injuries following penetrating scrotal injuries. This may include damage to the femoral vessels, bowel and bladder. Surgical exploration is indicated to identify the extent of any scrotal injuries and in severe cases orchidectomy may be required.

Skin Loss (Burns, Fournier's Gangrene)

Fournier's gangrene is a necrotising fasciitis of the perineum. A high index of suspicion must be maintained in any patient who presents with a scrotal/perineal cellulitis, particularly if they are diabetic. Patients with Fournier's present with sepsis and examination may reveal local signs of erythema, crepitus and skin necrosis. Urgent resuscitation, broad spectrum antibiotics and prompt surgical debridement are essential although despite this the mortality remains high. The primary focus for infection is often in the ischiorectal fossa/peri-rectal region and extensive debridement with urinary and/or faecal diversion may be required. Plastic and general surgical input is often needed. A re-look at 48 h is important to ensure that all diseased tissue has been removed. Testicles can be protected in a thigh pouch prior to eventual reconstruction using skin grafts and flaps.

Approximately 5–13 % of burns affect the external genitalia [6]. Scrotal skin has characteristics which enable good healing and as such most burns can be managed conservatively. Thermal burns are most commonly first or second degree although an insensate burn suggests deeper damage and may require debridement. Burns to the glans heal best via secondary intention [7].

References

1. Morey AF, Metro MJ, Carney KJ, Miller KS, McAninch JW. Consensus on genitourinary trauma: external genitalia. BJU Int. 2004;94:507–51.
2. Jezior JR, Brady JD, Schlossberg SM. Management of penile amputation injuries. World J Surg. 2001;25:1602–9.
3. Jordan GH, Jezior JR, Rosenstein DI. Injury to the genitourinary tract and functional reconstruction of the urethra. Curr Opin Urol. 2001;11:257–61.
4. Allen F, Morey AF, Dugill DD. Genital and lower urinary tract trauma. In: Campbell-Walsh urology. Wein AJ, Kavoussi LR, Novick AC, et al. editors. 9th ed. Philadelphia: Saunders Elsevier; 2007.
5. Lupetin AR, King W, Rich P, et al. The traumatized scrotum: ultrasound evaluation. Radiology. 1983;148:203–7.
6. Michielsen D, Van Hee R, Neetens C, LaFaire C, Peeters R. Burns to the genitalia and the perineum. J Urol. 1998;159:418–9.
7. Wessels HB. Genital skin loss: unified reconstructive approach to a heterogenous entity. World J Urol. 1999;17:07–14.

.

Chapter 21
Enterovesical Fistulae and Pneumaturia

Nicholas Raison and Ben Challacombe

Enterovesical fistulae (EVF) and the pathognomonic features of pneumaturia, faecaluria and recurrent urinary tract infections (UTI) were first described by Cripps in 1888 [1]. Defined is "an abnormal communication between the intestine and the bladder" [2], EVF represent a rare but devastating complication of advanced inflammatory and malignant disease or iatrogenic or traumatic injuries. Pneumaturia is the passage of air per urethram at the time of voiding and is the classic symptom of an underlying enterovesical fistula.

The most common aetiology is diverticular disease accounting for 50–70 % of cases. Malignancy, most commonly colorectal cancer, and inflammatory bowel disease account for a further 20 and 10 % of cases respectively. However the incidence of disease is low, occurring in 1–4 % of patients with diverticular disease and 0.5 % of patients with colorectal cancer. Fistulae can complicate surgical and endoscopic

N. Raison (✉)
Department of Urology, Guy's and St. Thomas'
NHS Foundation Trust, London, UK
e-mail: nicholasraison@googlemail.com

B. Challacombe, MS, FRCS (Urol)
Department of Urology, Guy's and St. Thomas' NHS
Foundation Trust, Great Maze Pond, London SE1 9RT, UK

B. Challacombe, S. Bott (eds.), *Diagnostic Techniques in Urology*,   185
DOI 10.1007/978-1-4471-2766-6_21,
© Springer-Verlag London 2014

procedures of the gastrointestinal (GI) and urinary tracts. They can also be caused by pelvic radiotherapy or foreign bodies (fish bones, gallstones and catheters have all been implicated).

EVF occur most commonly in the fifth and sixth decades with a significant male preponderance given the protective the interposition of the uterus between the bladder and bowel.

Fistulae can be classified into four categories based on their anatomical location; colovesical, rectovesical, ileovesical, and appendicovesical. Whilst colovesical are the most common, rectovesical are seen most frequently following surgery (e.g. radical prostatectomy). Fistulae can be further subdivided by their structure. Simple fistulae are smaller with single tracts found in non-irradiated or inflamed tissue. In contrast complex fistulae are larger, comprise multiple tracts and occur in the presence of irradiated tissue, colonic abscesses or obstructions.

Diagnostic Algorithm for Enterovesical fistulae

Investigation of suspected enterovesical fistula should confirm the presence of a fistula, delineate the anatomical location and structure of the fistula and finally establish the underlying pathology.

Clinical Examination

Although the causes of EVF are usually gastrointestinal in origin, patients most frequently present with urological symptoms. High bladder compliance together with low intravesical pressure favour flow from the bowel to the bladder. Pneumaturia and faecaluria are therefore far more common than urine flow from the rectum.

History

Up to 75 % of patients present with the pathognomonic symptoms of pneumaturia, faecaluria and recurrent UTIs [3]. However they may occur intermittently so should be carefully elicited in the history. Pneumaturia occurs in 60 % of patients and although there are other causes its presence should always arouse high levels of suspicion for a fistula. It is important to exclude other causes such as recent bladder instrumentation, emphysematous cystitis or pyelonephritis, UTI with gas forming organisms (e.g. *E. coli, Klebsiella pneumonia, Proteus,* and *Clostridium*) and yeast fermentation in diabetic urine.

But more generic urinary tract and bowel symptoms are also common at presentation and may obscure the diagnosis. Lower urinary tract symptoms of frequency, urgency, suprapubic pain and haematuria are frequently reported. Likewise lower GI symptoms such as a change in bowel habit, haematochezia (blood per anus), urinary flow via the rectum, diarrhoea and abdominal pain. Gouverneur's syndrome, a hallmark of EVF, is characterised by suprapubic pain, frequency, dysuria and tenesmus. A full medical history must also be taken to assess for possible causative aetiologies.

Examination

Physical examination is unlikely to determine the presence or location of a fistula; physical signs are generally limited to abnormal urine analysis, malodorous urine, debris in the urine or uncommonly signs of systemic sepsis.

A full examination should be conducted assessing for signs of inflammatory and neoplastic or other underlying disease.

Laboratory Investigations

Blood analysis is seldom helpful in diagnosis.

Urine analysis usually reveals bowel organisms and debris, most frequently E Coli and enterococci.

Urine centrifugation can show faecal or vegetable matter and cytology can reveal smooth muscles cells from the intestine.

To aid diagnosis a number of bedside tests can be performed. Ingestion of oral colouring agents such as charcoal with subsequent charcoaluria are up to 100 % sensitive in establishing the presence of a fistula. Likewise the poppy seed test, where poppy seeds are ingested and the urine analysed after 24–48 h is similarly effective [4].

Imaging

Plain abdominal radiography is rarely helpful although an erect film may reveal an air fluid level within the bladder. Contrast studies such as barium enemas and cystography have a limited use in the diagnosis of EVF but may be helpful in diagnosis of the causative disease.

Computerised tomography (CT) is the imaging modality of choice for the diagnosis of EVF [4]. Common findings include gas in the bladder (in the absence of recent instrumentation), oral contrast seen in the bladder in the absence of intravenous contrast and adjacent areas of bowel and bladder thickening. Three-dimensional reconstruction further improves the diagnostic capabilities through improved visualisation of the relationship the bladder to neighbouring structures.

Magnetic resonance imaging (MRI) offers a number of advantages over CT imaging [5]. It provides detailed soft tissue resolution in addition to multi-planar imaging capabilities. Furthermore fluid within the fistula acts a natural luminal contrast obviating the need for administration of an enteral contrast agents which can give false positive results if there is significant bowel oedema. Fistulae are seen as high signal tracts on T_2 weighted images whilst T_1 weighted images can delineate the extension of fistula relative to neighbouring viscera and local inflammation. The major limitations of MRI are the lack of availability in the acute and emergency setting and high cost.

Endoscopy

Cystoscopy is a vital component of the investigative algorithm for enterovesical fistula. It can both identify the location of a fistula within the bladder and exclude bladder pathology. Early signs include areas of localised oedema and congestion which develop into bullous oedema and mucosal hyperplasia.

On the other hand the main role for GI endoscopy (e.g. sigmoidoscopy and colonoscopy) is in identifying underlying bowel pathology. It has a low sensitivity for detecting fistulae and is used primarily to evaluate the bowel lumen; essential if colonic malignancy is suspected.

Management

EVF are challenging to manage and successful treatment relies on the accurate and timely identification of the fistula and diagnosis of the underlying pathology.

Following a focussed history and examination, all patients presenting with suspect EVF should undergo urine analysis (microbiology, centrifugation, cytology). The charcoal or poppy seed tests may be helpful in supporting the diagnosis but CT with contrast should be the first line imaging modality. Cystoscopy is routinely used to localise the fistula. MRI should be used as second line imaging if CT images are not conclusive. Concurrently the underlying aetiology should be investigated.

Treatment of EVF needs to be tailored to the patient and is highly dependent on the location of the fistula and underlying pathology. Options range from conservative management to endoscopic and laparoscopic or open surgical procedures.

Conservative management is generally reserved for patients unfit for surgery and is generally associated with a high morbidity.

Surgery (endoscopic, laparoscopic or open) remains the main stay for treatment of EVF. Endoscopic treatment is generally reserved for small iatrogenic perforations (<1 cm) and bowel stenosis treated with self expanding bare metal stents.

Laparoscopic and open surgery aims to resect the fistula and restore continuity (as either a primary or staged procedure). Defunctioning surgery is limited to high risk and palliative patients.

References

1. Cripps H, St Bartholomew's Hospital. Passage of gas and feces through the urethra; colotomy; recovery; remarks. Lancet. 1890;132(3396):619–20.
2. Scozzari G, Arezzo A, Morino M. Enterovesical fistulas: diagnosis and management. Tech Coloproctol. 2010;14(4):293–300. doi:10.1007/s10151-010-0602-3.
3. Holroyd DJ, Banerjee S, Beavan M, Prentice R, Vijay V, Warren SJ. Colovaginal and colovesical fistulae: the diagnostic paradigm. Tech Coloproctol. 2012;16(2):119–26. doi:10.1007/s10151-012-0807-8.
4. Kavanagh D, Neary P, Dodd JD, Sheahan KM, O'Donoghue D, Hyland JMP. Diagnosis and treatment of enterovesical fistulae. Colorectal Dis. 2005;7(3):286–91. doi:10.1111/j.1463-1318.2005.00786.x.
5. Ravichandran S, Ahmed HU, Matanhelia SS, Dobson M. Is there a role for magnetic resonance imaging in diagnosing colovesical fistulas? Urology. 2008;72(4):832–7. doi:10.1016/j.urology.2008.06.036.

Index

B. Challacombe, S. Bott (eds.), *Diagnostic Techniques in Urology*, 191
DOI 10.1007/978-1-4471-2766-6,
© Springer-Verlag London 2014